THE WIN-WIN OUTCOME

THE WIN-WIN OUTCOME

The Dealmaker's Guide to
Buying and Selling Dental Practices

BERNIE STOLTZ & MARK MURPHY

ISBN: 978-1-7328573-9-1
LCCN: 2018957376

Cover design by Jennifer Chevalier
Layout design by Wesley Strickland

I want to dedicate this book to my sons, Lucas and Bennett Murphy, who inspire me every day to be my best and constantly surprise me with their intelligence, kindness, and wisdom. I'm also grateful for the opportunity to be part of Fortune Management, which continues to be a vehicle to change the lives of doctors, their families, and their staffs all over North America.

–Mark Murphy

I want to dedicate this book to the support and growth of private practitioner dentistry in North America and to the hard working men and women of Fortune Management and their dedication to helping doctors turn their dreams into their realities for the last 30 years.

–Bernie Stoltz

TABLE OF CONTENTS

HOW M&A CREATES WINS FOR YOU, YOUR PATIENTS, AND YOUR NET WORTH

The dental profession has changed enormously over the last thirty years. The consumer has changed, corporate dentistry has grown, and private practitioners must adapt to a business environment vastly different from that of just a few decades ago. There's a lot that dentists need to consider about the future of their profession.

What do dental consumers want today? They want better and faster dentistry. They also want more affordable and more convenient dentistry. Over the last decade, the evolution of dentistry has gone into hyperspeed. The practices that remain on the cutting edge will be positioned for lasting success. The ones that don't will see their profitability continue to erode.

Thirty years ago, MDs began to form group practices or went to work for bigger health-care providers. This is the direction dentistry is heading in today. The evolution is underway, and it's not a choice; it's simply the reality of where the profession is going. Many dentists still operating under an older model may greet this change with fear. This is understandable. We wrote this book to help you get past that fear, because the future of dentistry offers enormous opportunities for dentists to run better practices, lead better lives, and create lasting wealth.

Private-practitioner dentistry has typically been one dentist working in his or her own practice four days per week. In this model, the average dentist in America today generates top-line collections of about $800,000 per year, with a 72 percent operating overhead. This means that a typical dentist is making $200,000 to $225,000 annually before taxes. One challenge with this model is the high overhead for a single doctor to manage; another challenge is that this model no longer matches what the modern dental consumer wants. With the number of millennials—the dominant sector of the workforce and population—having reached over 75 million, we know that consumer demand has changed.

Dentists have long been known to work four-day weeks, and to be home for dinner every evening. Yet a dental practice that is open four days a week, mornings and afternoons only, is not offering convenient care for most dental consumers, and corporate dentistry has risen to fill this void. Convenience has become a big part of marketing for dental practices, and many consumers are gravitating to the corporate model because of the convenience it offers.

More consumers are heading to corporate shops because those shops have zeroed in on what the consumer wants. The easiest hygiene appointments to sell in metro areas today are six, seven, and eight o'clock at night. Consumers today are looking for practices with extended hours, where insurance is accepted and payment plans are available, and where top-notch care is delivered with modern technology and multiple specialists under one roof.

As executive coaches at Fortune Management and Sequoia Private Client Group, one of our definitions of success is understanding what people want and how they want it, and then filling that need quickly and effectively. If you're in business today, you'd better find out what's most important to your customers and how to deliver it—and then deliver it really, really well.

In other words, fall in love with the customer. That's what corporate dentistry has been able to do. We recently surveyed ten thousand new dental patients with the help of 1-800-DENTIST, a marketing company that matches patients with dentists in their area, and we narrowed down the top reasons a new patient would choose one dental practice over another:

- Customers expect the practice to be in network with their insurance carrier.
- Customers want to be able to see a dentist in the evening or on a weekend.
- Customers want the practice to have modern technology.
- Customers want different specialists all under one roof. They don't want to go somewhere else to see an orthodontist or oral surgeon.
- Customers care about online reviews and a dental practice's website.

Customers care about affordability and flexibility of payment plans. When we looked at this picture, we thought, "Corporate dentistry is nailing it."

Now, let's compare what today's dental consumer wants with what the typical dental practice has been doing for the last thirty years: four days a week, typically Monday through Thursday, and limited hours—maybe thirty-two patient-exposure hours a week. Many practices don't want to participate in insurance or put together payment plans. It's just one solo practitioner working alone with a small team.

When we talk about evolving from that older model and adapting to today's environment, it's clear that dentists must be willing to merge. To compete in the new millennium, we're going to need to have multiple private practitioners working multiple shifts in state-of-the-art facilities. Together, private doctors can not only compete with corporate dentistry, but they can surpass it. Borrowing some strategies from the corporate model—such as extended hours, modern technology, and multiple specialists under one roof—allows private practitioners to flourish in this environment.

When doctors form group practices, if the merger is done properly, the result is higher quality and more convenient care for patients, and more money and better quality of life for the doctors. Associate, mid-career, and late-career doctors can all benefit from merging their practice with another. The evolution of dentistry has an enormous upside for any doctor with an entrepreneurial bent—and this is true for those who just want to grow their practices and for those who are looking to retire soon.

When both parties' interests are aligned, a practice employing two or more doctors under one roof is positioned for far greater profitability and success. This does not mean that we're aiming to turn the whole profession into corporate dentistry. Far from it. Private doctors can merge into a much more efficient business model without giving up their private-practitioner status or the opportunity to build equity in a practice. You're going to be able to provide patients with the same uncompromising standard of care they've always known and loved.

Twenty years ago, most of the deals we were doing were for doctors who were at or near retirement. Now, it's often the case that a younger doctor may be a great clinician but not a great business person; he or she doesn't know how to grow. Say that doctor has a smaller practice that might be doing $400,000–$700,000 a year. Unfortunately, with the associated overhead, that doctor is not putting a lot of money on the bottom line. He or she would be far better off—and would make more money—selling the practice to another clinician who's more entrepreneurially focused.

There is no better way for an entrepreneurial doctor to create wealth than to merge his or her practice with another. This is true regardless of whether you are a late-career dentist looking for a tax-efficient exit strategy and liquidity event or an entrepreneurial dentist who is just getting started.

Merging under one roof creates economies of scale—i.e., more dentistry output with limited additional costs. For example, a dentist with a $1 million practice is probably taking home around $300,000. By showing that dentist how to buy another $1 million practice, we can ensure that 40 percent of the money goes to the bottom line with little to no risk. Now, that doctor who was making $300,000 is making $700,000. You've got the revenue from two practices coming in with the fixed overhead of one facility. Neither the selling doctor nor the acquiring doctor has to spend more time turning a handpiece—and in some cases it's much less time for both doctors.

Keep in mind that it doesn't always have to be a sale. The future of dentistry is to practice in groups. If you take two practices each doing a million dollars a year and merge them properly, one plus one does not equal two in that equation. You take two million, put it under one roof with one staff, one fixed set of costs, and great coaching, and both doctors make more. It's not just about acquisitions or sales; mergers are going to be a big part of dentistry's future as well.

Being Consumer Friendly

To understand where dentistry is heading, it's also important to consider that dental practices are part of the retail arm of health care. Like veterinary medicine, plastic surgery, and optometry, dentistry is elective health care—in other words, services that aren't necessarily covered by insurance. Therefore, these practices need to be treated as a retail environment—more akin to Neiman Marcus than a brain surgeon's practice in an office building. Today, we're bringing dental facilities out to Main Street. We're building them in shopping centers nationwide. We're installing them in strip malls and other high-visibility retail environments because we want to be as consumer friendly as possible.

Thirty years ago, a dentist was extremely reliant upon his clinical skills. If a doctor had strong clinical skills and could offer an expensive menu of services, that doctor could build a profitable business. It is not that clinical skills are not still very important—they are, of course—but it is much, much more important today that doctors choose the right environment in which to practice. By environment we mean the technology, the office design and feel, and the team that surrounds the doctor.

We know that good technology in a good environment makes a dental practice more profitable and care more affordable, but it's expensive for a single practitioner. If you're going to invest in a million dollars' worth of technology, a high-visibility, high-profile location, and the best, most experienced team, it makes zero sense for a single doctor to use a facility only four days a week. We need to have a team of doctors using that facility six to seven days a week. The resulting increase in revenue will enable your merged practice to invest in higher-dollar technology than one single practitioner can afford on his or her own.

Most dentists were promised in dental school that they were going to work four days a week and be highly successful. Our system is about working less—as part of a team of doctors—and earning more. If you've got two dentists who each want to work three days a week, then between the two of them they're able to offer their patients six days of care a week. This allows for more comprehensive care, more convenience for the consumer, and a better life balance for each doctor.

Dentists are plagued with the same problem that all highly paid professionals have. Whether it's an attorney, an MD, an architect, a CPA, or a dentist, they all have the ability to command a high hourly wage. The challenge, though, is that the minute a doctor stops treating a patient or a dentist puts down a handpiece, he or she stops making money.

Making the Switch to Business Owner

So what dentists are really doing—what the whole profession has been doing up until now—is trading time for dollars. Most dentists think as clinicians, not as businesspeople, so they trade their time for a paycheck. But an entrepreneurial dentist asks, "How can I develop a practice that can make money while I sleep? How can I create a practice that will function even if I'm not there?"

One of the key challenges we want to put to our readers is this: Do you want to continue to be a business operator and a well-paid professional, or do you want to start making the shift to business owner? There's a big difference between an operator and an owner: An operator has to be there to get paid. An owner does not.

Dental school for most dentists is 95 percent or more about developing clinical skills. Yet the minute they graduate, enter the real world, and decide to go into private practice, that 95 percent of their dental education only accounts for about 33 percent of their overall success in private practice. They have to master the other two-thirds of the equation—one-third being business systems and business acumen, and one-third being communication and leadership skills. The right coaching will enable you to master those skills you didn't learn in dental school.

Again, we don't ever want to downplay the importance of our clients' clinical skills. What we're appealing to is your entrepreneurial spirit and your desire to create a better quality of life for yourself and provide better care for your patients.

When we're on the road giving talks to doctors around the country, we often refer to what we call a **Class 3 Experience**. This is an experience that's good for the patients, good for the practice, and good for the profession. When we take two practices and put them together, the patient wins because it means there's a more profitable business able to provide a better environment with modern equipment and multiple providers.

Who else wins? The practice wins, because it's now a more efficient practice positioned for steady growth. The doctors—the owners and partners—win because they now have a thriving, better practice. Finally, we're also benefiting the profession overall—it's a Class 3 Experience. And ultimately the staff wins as well, because they're now part of a growing business, not one that's treading water.

What's Important to You?

Is it taking care of the patients who have trusted you for many years? Is it looking after key staff members who have been loyal and helped you build your business? Is it making a graceful transition to retirement so you can work as much or as little as you want for the balance of your career? Is it about getting out immediately?

Every doctor is different, so we go through a process of finding out what's important to each doctor and then creating a plan to achieve each doctor's goals. Some of the most successful doctors we have don't turn a handpiece at all, or they do so only on a part-time basis. Of course, if they want to continue to work full time, they can do that.

Our clients seek to serve people and make the world a better place. An adage we tell many dentists is, "It's OK to do well at doing good things." That's what this book is about. We will show you how to be great at what you do, how to do a better job for your patients, how to do it in a great environment with great people, and how to deliver a truly high-quality product. At the same time, we're hoping to instill a mindset that says, "Hey, it's okay for us to do well financially."

The following chapters will help you understand practice sales and mergers in this new era of dentistry. We'll discuss why building, merging, or selling makes sense for you, and how we go about the process. We'll talk about why we take a customized approach to every deal so no two are ever the same. We'll look at creating a plan that combines your business, financial, and life goals. We'll look at how to prepare a practice for sale, how to determine the value of a practice you seek to buy or sell, and how to finance the purchase. We'll also look at the practice management strategies we use to turbocharge practices both before and after a merger or sale. Finally, we'll end by telling you how we create multigenerational wealth in dentistry, and invite you to continue the conversation with us.

Today, a pair or more of doctors can build a lucrative group practice that provides superior care for the consumer, the best environment for the staff, and a stable nest egg for each doctor. When an M&A is done properly, with creativity and synergy, it leads to a win-win outcome.

Chapter 1

HOW YOU CAN GROW, MERGE, OR SELL YOUR PRACTICE . . . RIGHT NOW

Whether you are looking to build, merge, or sell your dental practice, you have an opportunity to increase profitability and your standard of care. Corporate dentistry has changed the game, and we want to give you the tools to not only compete with corporate shops but outperform them.

When we sit down and talk to any doctor, even one who is getting ready to retire, almost invariably they want to grow their business because they want to sell it for more money upon retirement. The way they think they're going to grow is by getting more of the right kinds of patients in the chair, by doing great work, and by using both internal and external marketing techniques. They add one new patient at a time by getting current patients to refer their families, friends, coworkers, and neighbors.

However, a more efficient way to grow is to do it in one fell swoop by acquiring patients from another practice and moving them to your facility. Get those patients in the base first, then use various levers to turbocharge that practice—strategies such as increasing patient reactivation rates, offering a wider variety of advanced dental procedures, and securing higher reimbursements from insurance companies (we'll discuss these in chapter 11, "Turbocharging Your Newly Bought or Merged Practice"). There are lots of strategies to make a practice more profitable, not only for the buying doctor, but for the selling doctor as well.

In the model of doctor-as-business-operator, there is a limit to how much money you can make in a practice and how successful that practice can be. As we said in the introduction, we want doctors to make the shift from being business operators to being business owners. In addition to our various turbocharging strategies, we help doctors become leaders—not just managers of their practices, but leaders.

We want doctors to get paid for what they know, not what they do, because no matter how great a doctor is, there are only so many hours in a day and only so many years a doctor can practice dentistry. In every dental business, no matter how skilled the doctor is as a surgeon and marketer, there's tons of room for improvement. There is no such thing as perfect, and even if there were, you'd still be limited by the fact that you're only human. You could fall down a ski slope and find yourself out of work for six months. And even if you manage to avoid accident or injury, there is the inexorable march of time: as any doctor ages, his or her health inevitably becomes a factor.

To guard against this vulnerability, we want dentists to think of themselves not just as dentists, but as entrepreneurs with a specialty in dentistry. With this approach, even when a dentist's skills start to fade because of age, or when they simply become interested in spending less time chairside, their practice continues to pay them in multiple ways.

Here's a question: Do you want to play on the football team or do you want to own the team? Better yet, if you can do both, why not do both? If you want to play it like everybody's always played it before, we'll show you strategies that will enable you to do it better so you'll bring in a lot more income. But if you have an entrepreneurial bent, we want to get you to a place where you're not in the practice of dentistry, but in the business of dentistry. Now you own the team.

Ideally, we want every one of our clients to get paid four ways: as the landlord, as the doctor, as the CEO, and as the owner of a business. If after getting paid as the landlord and the doctor they are not putting at least 20 percent to the bottom line—and some of the best practices put 30 or 35 percent to the bottom line—they have not bought themselves a business; they've bought a well-paying job. However, a doctor who is putting 20 percent to the bottom line could, in theory, not turn a handpiece at all and still have a very profitable business that would earn him income for the rest of his life.

Whether you work chairside seven days a week for the next forty years or you never turn a handpiece again, we recommend that you get involved in the business of dentistry. From an income perspective, an asset perspective, and a quality-of-life perspective, doing this will make your life better in every way. The move from business operator to business owner can happen with minimal upset to your life. It may add a little complexity, but the upside is too significant to pass up. Asserting more control over your business will allow you to be the author of your future.

Why Does Growing Make Sense for You?

Before we get into how we facilitate mergers and acquisitions, let's talk about why. Do you want to build a much bigger asset? Do you want to earn double, triple, or quadruple what you can as a single practitioner? Are you looking at the long term, thinking of when you start to get older, your back and knees get a little creakier, your hands get a little less steady, and your eyesight gets a little worse? Do you want the option of not having to work chairside full-time? Are you concerned that if you can't operate at peak efficiency every day, your patients won't be taken care of and your profits will take a hit?

Say you have a mature, single-practitioner practice that's growing modestly at 3 to 5 percent a year. Or maybe the practice is struggling and shrinking at 3 to 5 percent a year (unfortunately more common than not). With the single-doctor model, you're not only limiting your asset value and income, you're also limiting the opportunities for your staff. If your practice is treading water while the best practices out there are growing—by providing what consumers want, like top technology, multispecialty under one roof, and extended hours—your best people will be attracted to the opportunity to make more money and work for a practice that's growing.

Most doctors want to build a future not only for themselves, but also for their teams. A staff member of a practice that's shrinking may be wondering, "Why am I going to want to spend ten, twenty, or thirty years with you if you're not going to give me the best opportunity to grow in my career and make the kind of money I need to support my family?"

Expenses go up every year, so revenue must grow by 4 or 5 percent a year just to stay even. If a practice is treading water, how can the doctor continue to increase staff salaries without dipping into personal savings? How can that doctor afford the new technology that patients are demanding? The best solution is a group practice that takes advantage of economies of scale: with the overhead of one facility and limited additional costs, multiple doctors provide better care and generate more revenue.

How to Grow, Merge, or Sell—From Letter to Lunch

Now the how. How you can build, merge, or sell—right now. Remember, this can happen with minimal disruption to your life. Let's say our client is looking to buy another practice and merge it into their facility. We craft a letter that goes out every month to every practice in the client's area in which at least 75 percent of the patients would come to our client's office. In New York City, that might be seven or eight blocks; in Montana, it might be a hundred miles. How far that 75 percent goes depends on the area's geography.

Or it could be a reverse merger, in which our client buys another practice and moves their practice into that building because it's a better facility or location. In that case, we make sure that at least 75 percent of our client's patients would be willing to travel to the new office.

There is little risk in bringing the patients over. Why would patients who have been with you for twenty or thirty years not want to come to work with you in your new facility? Once we identify the practices near our client's where 75 percent of the patients would come to our client's office, our letter talks about the offer and what's special about the practice.

Fifteen or twenty years ago, a letter of this nature was rare. Now, with the advent of corporate dentistry and books like this one being written about mergers and acquisitions, they're becoming more common. So the next question is, if you received one letter from a corporate outfit and one from a private practitioner, what would make the latter more interesting? What would make you say, "I'd really like to speak to the person who wrote that letter"?

In order to catch another doctor's eye, your letter must convey what's special about you. A prospect will be asking, "Why would I want to sell my practice to you? Why would my patients want to come to you? What is unique and special about the way you do business?" We answer those questions and send that letter every month.

The second thing we do is reach out to the dental community—practice brokers, supply companies, dental consultants, dental CPAs, dental attorneys, etc.—and let them know we're in acquisition mode. We put the word out to the world.

The third step involves networking. Often, the doctors we contact have been in their communities for years. They know other doctors, and other doctors know them. So a dentist interested in forming a partnership picks up the phone and says, "Hey, Joe, have you done any thinking about your transition or exit strategy? I've got some ideas. Maybe we could do something better together than we could apart. Are you free for a cup of coffee or lunch next week?" On many occasions a doctor's staff has worked in other offices, and they have friends who are hygienists or assistants in other offices, so a doctor in acquisition mode might tell his or her staff, "Hey, if you can introduce me to a practice that we close a transaction on and buy, I'll give you a $5,000 bonus."

Once we get somebody who has responded to the letter and agreed to a meeting, it's a straightforward process. We ask powerful, open-ended questions. We learn from that doctor what's important to them: Is it quality of care for the patients who have trusted them for many years? Is it taking care of key staff people? Maybe it's trying to get out from underneath some of the administrative work and just focus on dentistry. Is it exiting at their peak, so instead of letting things atrophy and selling the practice for a fraction of what it's worth, they can sell it at its highest value? Or maybe a doctor has a child, and while they still need to be a dentist two or three days a week, they also want more time at home with the baby. What's important to them could be any one of a thousand different concerns.

With clear goals laid out on both sides, we can then craft a win-win deal. The key to our approach is collaboration and synergy: Instead of win-lose, it's win-win—a collaborative, cooperative process in which both buyer and seller are getting exactly what they want. Our role is to help both sides see what's important to them, and then come back with a transition plan in place that gets everybody what they want. Nearly 100 percent of our deals end up closing because both parties are invested: What's important to each side is directly factored in. Very few doctors end up rejecting a plan that they themselves helped create.

Collaborative Deals

Chapter 7, "Making the Deal Work for Both Sides," will go into greater detail about how we achieve a win-win outcome for both sides, but we want to discuss it briefly here. If a transition plan doesn't have buy-in from both sides—if it's a cookie-cutter plan that says, "Here's the plan, take it or leave it"—then you can end up with a win-lose, or even a lose-lose. A cash walkaway sale requires a much higher level of due diligence because you're borrowing money and putting yourself on the hook.

We got into this business because we were saddened to see doctors who had worked their tails off for decades leave the profession with cash walkaway sales that paid them pennies on the dollar, with zero potential for creating lasting wealth—barely enough, in fact, to sustain them in retirement. We also saw doctors get involved in poorly orchestrated transition plans that didn't address what was truly important to them.

To make sure that each doctor gets what they want, we put together deals in a collaborative manner. Forming collaborative partnerships makes for healthier practices. Until the buyout is completed, doctors merging their practices are going to be partners in that new business. Even if the selling doctor is staying on as an associate, they're going to be partners for at least five years. So the best attitude to take toward this partnership is, "Let's work together and grow this thing as much as we can, because we're both positioned to benefit."

You want to end the relationship as friends and partners, and that means you want to start the relationship with a partnership in which each side is working hard to make sure the other party does better, because it will help them directly.

That's the magic of the win-win outcome, as opposed to a cash walkaway sale: synergy. We're big believers in an earn-out for either the entire deal or a large percentage of it. Then both parties' interests are aligned; the growth of the newly merged practice directly benefits both sides. (We'll cover how we finance deals in chapter 10, "How to Finance the Purchase or Sale of a Practice.")

For a doctor who owns a practice, it's all about profitability. Again, we want our clients to get paid four ways: as landlords, doctors, CEOs, and owners. An entrepreneurial dentist with the right dental coach can look at all kinds of opportunities—even merging with a practice that has been underperforming. An excellent executive coach can take a moderately profitable practice and make it wildly profitable with a few turbocharging strategies.

Attorney Involvement

When bringing a deal to fruition, each side has an attorney. One of the attorneys drafts an agreement that includes everything both sides have agreed to. Selecting attorneys is important. You need the right attorneys—not mercenaries who are there to run up legal bills or fight unnecessarily, but two attorneys who say, "Look, both parties agree that this deal puts them in a better position than they are now.

Let's figure out a way to put this down on paper at a reasonable cost and get this deal moving."

We help our clients find forward-thinking business attorneys who are not only familiar with mergers and acquisitions but who also have specific knowledge of dentistry and how these transactions play out in the dental world. We are always happy to work with a client's attorney, but keep in mind a few reasons why we believe the attorneys involved should have specific knowledge of dentistry.

First, dentistry is a unique animal: Typically, practices are sold based on gross earnings rather than EBITDA (Earnings Before Interest, Tax, Depreciation and Amortization, a measure of a company's operating performance), which is different from how most businesses are sold. Basing a sales figure on EBITDA means higher practice valuation (more on this in chapter 6, "Determining the Value of the Practice You Seek to Buy or Sell"). Second, there are licensing issues. You can't sell a practice to someone who's not a licensed dentist; it's not a doughnut shop or a car wash. The third reason is dental insurance. Some insurance carriers will pay a successor doctor as much as 40 percent less than they're paying the current doctor. You need to know about that in advance and plan accordingly—which means you need to have an attorney who understands these types of transactions.

One of the keys to creating real wealth is putting together a world-class team of attorneys, accountants, and bankers. You don't want to surround yourself with below-average—or even average—people. A world-class team works together like an orchestra, not like a group of random instruments. The wrong attorneys, instead of creating a sense of partnership, optimism, and opportunity, make the negotiations so torturous that by the time the deal is done the doctors are exhausted and angry. That's not what you want. A sale or merger means the doctors are going to be business partners for a while, perhaps for a long time, and you want to maximize the opportunity.

When you pick the right people, both parties come in soaring, excited by the opportunity, and the deal gets done quickly for a fair and reasonable fee.

Chapter 2

WHY NO TWO DEALS ARE
EVER THE SAME

Our approach—creating collaborative, win-win deals—focuses on what is important to each doctor involved. This is a customized process that must be undertaken for every client. Two practices that each do a million dollars of dentistry a year should not be treated the same. Some doctors aren't interested in turning a handpiece any longer, whereas some still want to be chairside four days a week. We always begin with what matters to each doctor. All doctors have different approaches and different concerns, and in twenty years we haven't had two deals that were exactly the same.

After we get clear on everything that is important to one side, we always say to the other side, "We can get everything we want by helping the other side get what they want first." The art of dealmaking is collaboration, rather than negotiation that causes one side to lose so the other can win. We sit down and work on it. Focusing on synergy, our process facilitates the best deal and best working partnership.

In many cases, those doctors are going to be partners for at least five years; at that point each party can walk away with a lot more money than if they had just done a cash walkaway sale or if the nego-tiation had been adversarial rather than collaborative.

The interesting thing about selling a dental practice is that there are very few rules. This allows us a lot of freedom to structure deals how we want. We don't craft cookie-cutter, one-size-fits-all deals. We make each deal based on the circumstances, needs, and desires of each of the doctors, then facilitate a transaction that advances each doctor's interests. We can get everything we want by helping other people get what they want, too.

Point A to Point B

Every doctor has them. Coaching doctors through a sale or merger begins with identifying these two points: Where are they now (point A), and where do they want to go (point B)? No two deals are equal because no two doctors start off in same place, nor are their endgames ever exactly the same.

If we've got somebody who is early to mid career—what we call the "growth phase"—and is moving toward the entrepreneurial model we talked about in the introduction and the first chapter, then we're going to want to sit down with them and ask, "Where are you right now?" This step requires due diligence on our part: We take a close look at their current profitability, lifestyle, and earning require-ments. It's a holistic approach, taking into consideration not just the value of their practice, but their current lifestyle and financial plan.

We go through that same process with the client who is looking to grow and the client who is looking for a liquidity event and maybe an exit strategy. We want to be very clear that it's not just about an exit strategy. We don't ever want to talk to somebody about retirement or selling a business or having a liquidity event until we are clear about the financial planning side of things. What are their needs going to be if they do not have that income coming in?

We always do a cash flow analysis for the selling doctor. A cash flow analysis takes into account everything else in the doctor's financial life besides their business. Once we complete that analysis, if the practice gets sold in the way we have laid out, that doctor will be able to have an abundant retirement. And they'll know exactly what that picture looks like before they sign away one of their most important assets—their practice.

Customizing the Deal = Win-Win

Once we've got clear points A and B from both sides, then the deal is customized. We figure out how we can make it so both parties win, and we have a great track record over the last twenty years of doing just that.

The key is to sit down with the two doctors and coordinate a deal once we know where everybody started, where each doctor is now, and where they want to go. Each customized deal creates a partnership where both parties do better.

The fun part for us is crafting that kind of deal. If that's not the case, why would we do this? We pride ourselves on never putting our names on a deal in which there's a clear winner and loser. We don't want to do that—ever. We would not want to be in a business in which for one side to win the other had to lose.

Sometimes a selling doctor wants to be a permanent associate. Sometimes that doctor wants to get out quickly. We may have an older doctor who's nearing the end of his or her career and has a sudden health problem that forces retirement. In this case, we'd need to figure out a proper transition to get that doctor out of the business as soon as possible.

If we can find out what's important to them, then the process becomes easy. Then we're able to start looking ahead. If this practice could be a stronger asset after it is sold, bought or merged, what's the next important goal? How is that going to make life better? How is that going to make the finances better? How is that going to bring the retirement goals closer?

Challenging Deals: Family Negotiations and Teardown Practices

We do a lot of family negotiations—situations in which a parent is passing on their practice to a son or daughter. Family dynamics can make this difficult. With family succession negotiations it's not just about the deal itself; it's about things like equalization among siblings. In these types of deals, we're not dealing only with a business; we're dealing with the family itself. We engineer deals so that they become projects all parties are working on together, with mutually beneficial outcomes.

Another challenge is working with clients whose practices are in decline. We travel around the country giving speeches to doctors, and in every audience in every city we have six or more teardown practice doctors who don't have a sellable asset. They're losing money, and in some cases they're actually draining retirement accounts to keep these failing businesses afloat.

In many cases, we've helped that sixty-five or seventy-year-old doctor to migrate their patient base into another practice operated by a young, mid-career dentist with a state-of-the-art facility.

There are thousands of older doctors out there who are considering retirement. Many would stay on, however, if they didn't have to run the business but could still treat their patients and do what they really love to do clinically. This process prolongs careers and in some cases it can prolong lives.

Remember that associate, mid-career, and late-career doctors can all benefit from M&As. Today, 50 percent of dental school graduates are female—the highest percentage ever. And many of them initially want to own their own practices. After a few years of running their own businesses, however, some discover that they want to pursue other dimensions of a balanced life, like being a mom, and being able to come home and cook dinner at five o'clock. Although they still have their love of dentistry, they don't necessarily have a love of business.

We work with all kinds of scenarios. Creating synergy gives doctors the opportunity to create more wealth and to have the lives they want.

Holistic Approach

In addition to being collaborative, our process is also all-inclusive. We cover every angle so the deal is synergistic from beginning to end. For example, as part of our holistic approach we address tax strategies, usually by bringing CPAs into the conversation. We also bring in legal counsel, and as we outlined in the last chapter, we work with attorneys who understand the unique animal that is dentistry.

But prior to bringing in attorneys, it's critical that both sides are on the same page. We'll say, "Look, we're not even going to bring the attorneys in until we all agree in principle on our desired outcomes and how we want to do this." We never allow attorneys to engage in adversarial negotiations.

Once you get into the weeds with each deal, there are many nuances. With some deals, the practice that's selling has zero debt on it. Other times, the practice has lots of debt, and that needs to be addressed. Does the debt need to be paid off before the transaction, or does the debt get acquired as part of the deal? Sometimes there are lease issues.

We're big advocates of every doctor having a professional entity, whether that be an S-Corp, a C-Corp, or an LLC. We're also big advocates of great tax strategies. In the income tax world, some deals benefit one side more than the other. For example, there are tradeoffs to paying taxes at capital gains rates. For one person to take a deduction, the other person has to declare income. We try to remind our clients that a dollar is not a dollar is not a dollar. A dollar is only the percentage, and that's all that you get to keep and put in your pocket. We want a holistic deal that maximizes our clients' tax payouts.

In many cases, in fact, we've encouraged our clients to accept less or to pay more because it was more tax advantageous. They could take the full deduction in the current year, rather taking the deduction over fifteen years. No deal works in a vacuum or a silo; that's why you have to know both sides' financial situations intimately.

There are many other moving parts as well: asset sales, stock sales, earn-outs, associate contracts—all kinds of levers we can pull for each doctor going into a sale or merger. Two basic functions that vary from deal to deal are what is paid for the buyout and what the doctor is paid for dentistry when they come to work as an associate. In these situations, you want to keep tradeoffs in mind: You may overpay a little for the practice, but you'll pay a smaller percentage on the associate work. Or maybe you pay a higher percentage for the associate work and less for the practice.

We once had a deal in which we sold the practice for zero dollars, but the clinician got 58 percent payout for as long as they worked. It's like the Marines: The skinny guys get strong and the fat guys get lean. There are twists and turns on virtually every deal, and that's why no two deals are done the same way.

For us, it's not only getting both sides what they want that makes each deal interesting. It's also the personalities. One of the things you learn when you work with dentists is that they are often very colorful characters. The art in our work is trying to craft a win-win deal for people who are very different from one another. Often, we're dealing with two doctors who are used to being the alpha in their practice. Each has different ideas and different quirks, and it's a challenge to make it work.

Our process is about simplicity. We need one initial meeting—a diagnostic meeting. Like dentists, we believe that diagnosis without an examination is malpractice, so we want to find out from the doctor how they think not just about their business, but about their money, their family, and their life. It's important for us to remember that money is never just math; it's always psychological. If you deal only with a client's money, you're only dealing with one of the factors that are important to them.

The second meeting may go a couple of hours or more. In that meeting, we lay out our recommendations and a clear strategy for going forward. By the end of that second meeting, in most cases it's clear whether the doctor should have a relationship with us or not. That is not done on a leap of faith; it's done by laying out a systematic way forward. It's essential to show that doctor a clear path. With a clear path, there's no leap of faith—the doctor is a partner in the plan.

Chapter 3

YOUR LIFE-PLAN EQUATION: CAREER PLAN PLUS FINANCIAL PLAN EQUALS HAPPINESS

In this chapter we're going to ask you, the reader, some questions. We're going to ask you to consider whether you've made good or bad career decisions up to now. This can be an enjoyable process or a painful one. Sometimes coaching is about putting people into pain points if that's what it takes to get them to take action, whether in the financial arena or any other area of life.

If you're a new client, right at the beginning we start a conversation about your life plan. We ask five questions: The first thing we want to know is where you are right now in your life and with your finances. Second, we want to know how you got there, and whether that is a great story or a nightmare.

Third and most important, we ask where you want to be—to tell us what that point B is. What if life in a year or five years or ten years was not just good, but great? Never settle for good: Good is the enemy of great. If your life were great, if you had power of purpose and could enjoy life to the fullest while helping everyone around you enjoy their lives to the fullest, if you lived by choice rather than doing things because you had to—what would that life look like?

We then ask you to define that clearly. Define it for your emotional state of mind. Define it for your physical health. Define it for your relationships. Define it for your spirituality, your connectivity to a higher power, or your ability to give back to the world. Define what your career would look like if you had total power of purpose. Define what your wealth would look like. We want to get really clear on where our clients want to be. You have to understand that money is not really what you want; what you want are choices, and money will get you choices.

The fourth question we ask is whether you have a plan in place to get yourself there." And the fifth is how we can help. If we've clearly delineated where you are now and where you want to get to, we can always come up with a strategy to get from point A to point B. That's what great coaches do.

* * *

Many dentists who are trading time for dollars allow that money to run their lives. We help our clients do the exact opposite: have the life they want now, keep it that way forever, and never run out of money. When we speak to dentists across the country, we talk about three different dimensions of any doctor's life: their lifestyle, their career, and their financial plan. Ultimately, we want to figure out how doctors can make the shift from trading time for dollars to being financially independent of work. This does not necessarily mean retirement. Rather, it means reaching a critical mass in their financial portfolio to create a blended annual rate of return that supports their current lifestyle whether they work or not.

In creating a life plan, what's important to them drives the process. What are their core values? What's possible? What should their lives be? Human beings—not just doctors, but all of us—have the tendency to get stuck in ruts. We forget that we have options and choices for how we want to live the rest of our lives. The old saying, "Keep your nose to the grindstone," is not always the appropriate approach. Sometimes it takes creative thinking to step outside the box and say, "I'm going to get very clear on what's important to me in my life and then work backwards from there. How does that affect my day-to-day life? What am I doing now for the life I want in the future?"

A lot of people doing practice sales, transitions, and mergers are trying to handle every practice the same way. The problem with that approach is that it's not about the individual doctor's goals. Some doctors love to practice dentistry. They're in their glory when they're holding a handpiece and have a patient in the chair. We also have mid- or late-career doctors who would like to do less dentistry, or no dentistry at all. There are a variety of reasons for this, including just the physical wear and tear on them as they age—they're tired and want to retire early.

We've developed strategies that allow you to practice less and make more money. Many dentists have the mindset that the only time a dentist is making money is when he or she is holding a drill, yet there are many different ways to make money. There are doctors making small fortunes with fee-for-service-only practices. Or with insurance practices. Or with HMO practices. Or with hybrids. There are many ways to achieve one's goals. What we want to do is open them up to the idea that everything is possible. Once everything is possible, the game slows down. Then you can really focus on what you want.

The question is, Where do you want to get? What's the end goal? Once we understand where we're going, we can reverse engineer from that endpoint in order to get there. This may involve running a cash flow analysis to determine what the business model needs to do in order for the client to reach his or her goals. The practice may need to grow in order to create economies of scale. There are many different directions it can go. But reverse engineering is the first step. A lot of business people—not just doctors—do not reverse engineer a plan for their businesses or their lives, and this is a mistake.

We encourage dentists to take a deep breath and really think about the future. Having worked with dentists at all career stages, from residents to doctors in their eighties, we've seen that a lot of the career and financial problems dentists have to solve in the second half of their careers are problems they created in the first half. They made decisions they would not have made if they had known where they wanted to end up. That's part of what we do: we help doctors get clear on where they want to be.

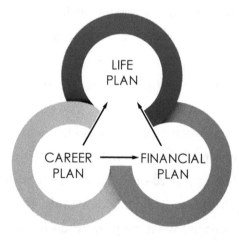

Three-Part Life Plan: Lifestyle, Career, Financial

We want you to be willing to take a 10,000-foot view of a whole life plan that focuses on three things: The first, which we put at the top of a pyramid, is what we call a lifestyle. Not just a life plan, but a lifestyle. With our help, most of the dentists we work with find a way to live a good lifestyle—a way to live in the homes they want to live in, drive the cars they want to drive, send their kids to the right schools, and take the vacations they want to take.

The lower left corner of the pyramid is the dentist's career plan. What is the career plan for the typical dentist? Traditionally, the career plan has been trading time for dollars. We've covered how dentists suffer from the same challenge as other well-paid professionals: MDs, attorneys, CPAs, and architects can all command a good hourly rate for their services, but few have learned to move from business operator to business owner. Remember the difference: a business operator has to be there to get paid, but a business owner makes money all the time.

A dentist's career plan has two moving parts: the doctor's practice and the execution of that business, which happens to be a dental practice. If we draw an arrow from the dentist's career plan to their lifestyle, we would see that their career plan—their practice—is supporting their lifestyle.

But that is not financial freedom. That is not financial independence. Financial independence consists of a financial plan that creates a critical mass in the doctor's portfolio to support their current lifestyle in perpetuity, whether they are working or not.

The lower right corner of the pyramid is the doctor's **financial plan**. With a critical mass invested in the doctor's money-making machine, just the annualized interest from those diversified asset allocations is enough to support the doctor's lifestyle without ever touching the principal.

At Fortune Management, we work with our doctors on an ongoing basis to make sure there's a financial plan in place that ultimately creates independence from working. When that is the case, you can draw an arrow from financial plan to lifestyle.

In other words, our client can still live in the same house, drive the same cars, fund the kids' and grandkids' educations, or whatever else they want to do, just as they could when they were working. The difference is that they are now doing it just from the annualized interest from their passive investments. This is how a dentist goes from trading time for dollars to financial independence—by building a critical mass in their portfolio so their money machine has a life of its own.

We want our clients to get very clear on what financial independence means. Few people fully grasp the concept and its implications. Today, most Americans are not able to retire with financial independence at age sixty-five or seventy. This is a challenge to society, and it's a social problem. We're not working on social problems in this book, of course, but we are working on helping dentists take care of themselves and their families.

Where Are You in This Conversation?

If you never worked again in your life, if you never held another handpiece, could you continue living the exact same lifestyle you're living right now while you're owning and operating your practice?

We aren't talking about downsizing your lifestyle or about selling your practice in New York and going to live in a two-bedroom condo in Boca. It doesn't mean changing how you live your life—how you eat, the vacations you take—because that's not what our clients want. They want a lifetime of financial freedom.

We hope to challenge you to look at your financial portfolio. Really take a look at it: Is the money invested correctly so that it is getting an aggressive annual rate of return? And are you clear about what your financial needs are? Have you done an inventory of your lifestyle, both as it currently sits and what it's going to look like five and ten years from now? That's the throw-down to the reader.

Three Ways to Wealth Creation

One of the things Fortune Management and Sequoia Private Client Group excel at is showing doctors how to create practices they don't even need to work in. This doesn't entail holding a handpiece more— or even at all. For a doctor's financial plan to work as intended and support the doctor's lifestyle in perpetuity, it must create wealth. Wealth creation is different from earning money by practicing your trade. Wealth creation is when more money is generated by the money itself, not by you.

Ultimately, there are three ways to be in the wealth creation business. The first is through the ownership of operating companies. This is an important one for our readers because most dentists either own a practice or want to own one, even if they're younger and just getting started in their careers. We want to emphasize that that practice is an operating company, and that is one of the first places we want to make sure they're making great investments. Your dental practice should be set up as an operating company whether you work in it and do dentistry or not. It's not something that necessarily needs to be sold at retirement time when you go into the financial independence phase.

A dentist knows no business better than the business of dentistry. Now, we could advocate for our clients to go out and buy an ice cream parlor or a car wash. Those are operating companies, too, but doctors probably don't know a lot about those businesses. They do know a lot about dentistry. They've got years of experience in and knowledge about the business. Therefore, our first move is always to maximize their investments in operating dentistry companies—which means their own practices, first and foremost, but also other practices.

There are other ways to invest in operating companies through 401(k)s, IRAs, or the open stock market. A dentist may be interested in taking an equity position in multiple companies in different industries. Regardless of which avenue they use, all of those come down to one segment of the dentist's portfolio: owning operating companies.

This kind of thinking is a paradigm shift for dentists. In our decades of experience working with executive coaching and practice management companies all over the country, the strategy has always been to build up the practice for twenty, thirty, or forty years and then do a cash walkaway sale. The problem with that strategy has always been that by the time a dentist has paid off the debt and taxes, they're walking away with a fraction of the money they need to support their current lifestyle in retirement.

Fortune and Sequoia together help doctors elongate their income-generating years. Rather than selling practices in their fifties and sixties, doctors are now buying practices in their sixties, seventies, and eighties because they've got decades of wisdom and experience, an entrepreneurial spirit, and great coaching. Backed by executive coaching from Fortune and wealth management from Sequoia, a dentist can make more money through passive ownership of dental practices than they were earning chairside in their early career.

We create multigenerational wealth for our clients not by trying to get out as soon as we can, but by keeping the ownership, flow of income, and tax benefits coming in perpetuity. Other businesses work this way, but this hadn't been done in dentistry until Fortune. You don't see the owner of a great manufacturing company say, "Hey,

I'm sixty-five years old—it's time to sell my business." No. Those businesses stay in the family for generations.

We understand that this is a paradigm shift, and it's not for every doctor out there. But for those who get it—and an awful lot of them do once you explain to them how it works—this is one of the biggest keys to creating multigenerational wealth.

For decades now, dentists have followed the strategy of build the practice, sell the practice, and take what you can get. Our question is, Why would a dentist spend all that time building a business and then sell it for pennies on the dollar?

Many doctors are still using this model because they've never set up a repeatable process. The process for generating earned income in perpetuity comes down to three things for every dental practice—culture, structure, and strategy. By creating excellence in those three areas, our clients don't have to continue to work inside their practices for them to be money-generating assets in their portfolio.

For our most successful doctors, there comes a tipping point where we feel we've put all our eggs in the dentistry basket. To spread the risk around, we're now seeing these doctors start to diversify their investment, operating companies not in the dental field. They act like operating businessmen. We generally don't take that step until we believe the client has hit a critical mass of investments in dental-related operating companies, but we're seeing more and more successful dentists getting to that point. When a dentist becomes a business operator, his or her core business is entrepreneurship. These doctors are entrepreneurs with a specialty in dentistry.

* * *

The second of three ways to get into the wealth creation business is through income-generating real estate. We help clients invest in real-estate opportunities that provide cash-on-cash return. This does not include a dentist's principal residence, however. It's vital to recognize that while they may have a lot of money in equity in their principal residence, while they are living there, that home is a liability. It's not an asset because it generates no money to support the doctor's lifestyle. If anything, it costs them money to live in that house.

So, what are income-generating real estate opportunities? First and foremost, we want to coach our clients, if it's appropriate, to own the real estate where their practices are. Whenever possible, we want our doctors to own the roofs over their heads. Those are income-generating pieces of property with guaranteed rents. Either they're going to pay rent to themselves from their company P&L if they continue to own it, or if they have partners or create an exit strategy they would continue to own that real estate in their portfolio, which again is passive income.

Because of the country's 1031 tax exchange laws, income-generating real estate is very portable. We want our clients to take a look at professional buildings. Maybe it's not just their practice but a whole building of doctors. Or maybe it's an apartment complex or single-family residences. Whatever the type of real estate, we want them pursuing investments in income-generating real estate.

The third way to wealth creation is being on the other side of the lending equation—being the bank, the VC, or the private equity. The higher net worth dentists whom we've worked with over the years have become the private equity to larger groups of dental practices. When they're on the lending side of the transaction, dentists can become a mini version of the investment banker or the private equity firm, able to take their capital and reinvest in other operating companies.

The bottom line is, if it's handled properly, we can put our higher net worth clients into private equity that invests predominately in dental practices where we can deliver them 20 percent cash-on-cash returns on an annual basis—on top of tax-free growth in the asset.

This doesn't mean the dentist is going to go out and open an investment bank. It doesn't mean they're going to be a venture capitalist to a software company. Those are probably not things most dentists want to be involved in. But we certainly want our clients to have well-balanced portfolios in the first two areas—owning operating companies and investing in income-generating real estate. If they are also interested in being on the lending side of the equation, we would want them looking at private equity ventures that had something to do with what they know.

* * *

At Fortune and Sequoia we bring clients through this entire process. Most dentists are able to maintain a great lifestyle while they're still holding a handpiece, but we can also give them, with a pretty high degree of certainty, a lifestyle that will last forever. We've got the tools and technology that get results—if the doctors are coachable—nearly 100 percent of the time.

Now, not every doctor wants to do all of what we've talked about. What's important to us is how that doctor thinks and what he or she is willing to do. The enjoyable part for us is getting to know who they are and what their objectives are—not our objectives but theirs—and then helping them achieve those objectives in an efficient way that's comfortable for them.

Paradigm Shift

Regardless of where you stand on the three wealth creation strategies, we are asking our readers to consider a paradigm shift. This is a new way for dentists to think about their careers, their businesses, and how they handle their practice transitions (an inevitable part of every dental practice and every business, which we'll talk about more in the next chapter, "Understanding the Life Cycle of a Dental Practice"). It is a psychological shift that has to happen. It's available to them, but they've got to value it and see that there's a different way of doing things than what dentists have typically done in the past—work until a certain age and then do a cash walkaway sale.

A paradigm shift in thinking does not come about easily. Some soul-searching is required. There has to be a powerful why for every doctor we work with. Why are you reading this book? Why would you want to consider this paradigm shift? Why would you want to hold onto your business into the future? Why would you want to build a critical mass in your portfolio? Most important, why do you want the lifestyle that you want?

Most strategies out there are not wealth creation strategies. The strategies most people adopt for practice sales and transitions are like the old Christmas club idea, which was to save all year so that in December you'd have money to buy Christmas presents for your family. You were earning about zero interest from the bank. It wasn't a wealth strategy, but more of a spending strategy.

The dental profession is by no means the only profession that suffers from this problem. In some other professions, it's even worse. Most MDs are told right when they get out of medical school that they'd better make all their money and fund their retirement plans while they're working, because at the end of that process they're going to hand their patients off, walk away, and not even have a resale event. The same goes for attorneys: hand off the clients and walk away. Very rarely does an attorney have a liquidity event when they leave a partnership. That is changing now, but the change must come from a paradigm shift in thinking. What we're here to do with this book is open some minds.

We have our clients figure out exactly what it's costing them right now, in 2018 dollars, to live their current lifestyle. What exactly is their house payment? What exactly is their car payment? We talk about the different levels of financial freedom and then ask our clients, in planning for your future, what other niceties of life would you like to add to your budget? Fully funding your child's education? A month in Italy? Whatever it is, let's get hard numbers so we know what our critical mass has to be in order to generate that lifestyle.

This is where the goal-setting process comes in for our clients. What if you had permission to dream big, to live better than you're living today without working in the future? If you were financially free from having to show up at the office every day, what would that life look like? What if, in the last twenty or thirty years of your life, you lived better than you're living now? You could live in a better location, you could give more to charity, and you could leave more to the next generation of your family. What if you could do more not working that you can currently do working—by building a money machine? And what if that money machine generated more wealth than you ever made by trading time for dollars?

Chapter 4

UNDERSTANDING THE LIFE CYCLE OF A DENTAL PRACTICE

Just like any other business, just like a human being or any other living thing, a dental practice has a life cycle. Just as a human being is born and goes through stages of development, so does a dental practice. In our talks around the country and directly with our clients, we always explain this life cycle. Whether doctors are early, mid, or late career, they need to be aware of certain stages and plan for how they will address them.

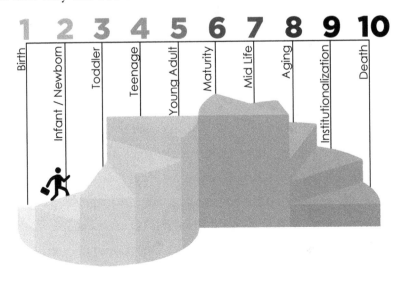

The ten life stages of a dental practice resemble a bell curve: birth, infancy, toddler, teenage, young adult, maturity, midlife, aging, institutionalization, and death. In this chapter, we want to make sure that readers are very clear about where their practice sits in that life cycle. Doctors whose practices are in the early years need to understand where their growth can come from, while doctors whose practices are aging need to realize that they have decisions to make. A bad decision is to do nothing, keep your head down, and just keep working as things continue to erode.

We also want dentists to be clear about where they are in their career life cycle. There are two life cycles we're concerned about—a practice life cycle and a career life cycle—and they are not necessarily the same.

Birth Through Teenage Years

Let's start with the practice life cycle. Dentists who have started from scratch have given birth to a business. That's no different from giving birth to a living entity. They've gone through some difficult growing stages, from infancy, through toddlerhood, and into the teenage stage. We always emphasize that the teenage stage of any business, including a dental practice, is by far the most dangerous time. This is very similar to a human teenager. We know that teenagers believe that they're going to live forever and that they're bulletproof. Often they take risks. Dentists with a teenager mentality are no different.

It's important for the reader to identify whether they're still in that teenager phase. Dentists with a teenager mentality still believe they can sell their way out of anything. They don't pay attention to cost overheads. They don't have an organized management structure. Unfortunately, what they do during the teenage stage is focus, all the time, on just selling more business. This is not just true of dental practices; many business owners think they can sell their way out of any problem. Sometimes they're interested in strategies, but they never work on the culture or structure of their business. All they do is chase the next big deal.

We've already talked about the three big things that are usually missing during the teenage phase of a dental practice: culture, structure, and strategy. The teenage-mentality dentist is just trading time for dollars and doesn't really have a plan for the future. Dentists often come to Fortune Management with this mindset: "Just help me get more patients, and everything will be fine. Show me how to market, and everything will be fine."

Not all teenage-mentality dentists are early in their careers. We've had doctors in their fifties and sixties who were still trying to sell their way out of every problem.

Zone of Maximization

Ultimately, any business should strive to be in the zone of maturity. Another term we use for this stage is zone of maximization. What defines the zone of maximization for a dental business? It's when a practice is most productive, most profitable, and 90 percent of the focus is on its patients and creating raving fans. That's what we want—the zone of maximization—and that's where we focus on taking all our dental practices.

However, as optimal a place as the zone of maximization is, it's also a precarious place that can lead quickly into midlife and aging. When a lot of dentists get to their zone of maturity they'll say, "Well, I don't know that it can get any better than where I am right now." Dentists who think they've gone as far as they can go need to realize that there's always another level.

At the top of the bell curve, there might be a whole other arc of growth for that business. A quote from Ray Kroc, the man who made McDonald's a household name, sums it up: "Are you green and growing or ripe and rotting?" Dentists in the zone of maximization who buy, sell, or merge through collaborative, win-win deals are positioned for another arc of growth.

Aging

The alternative to growing is aging ("ripe and rotting"). The aging decline includes four stages: midlife, aging, institutionalization, and death.

What does midlife look like for a dental practice? They've lost a notch. From the zone of maximization they've taken a step down the other side of the mountain. During midlife, which we also refer to as midlife crisis, they're not quite as profitable nor productive. Sadly, it's usually self-inflicted: they've been earning a healthy income and trading time for dollars, but now they want to spend it.

It's no different than a human being going through a midlife crisis. They start believing that they're past their prime, so they do things to reassure themselves that they've still got it. Now they want to take a three-week vacation in Europe instead of two. Now they want to make sure they golf every week. Now they're focusing on quality of life and life balance. The challenge, though, is that doctors whose practices are in midlife crisis haven't figured out how to have a sustainable life balance. They're still trading time for dollars. They have a professional paycheck, but they haven't built a company.

A midlife crisis practice is still making money but doesn't have a plan going forward. Dentists who were once in the zone of maximization but have not made the right decisions have left the maturity stage—they've come off the top of the hill—and are now in the midlife crisis stage and heading quickly into aging.

At that point doctors might tell themselves, "I'm just going to fund the hell out of my retirement plan, my 401(k), and whatever else I've got, and at some point I'm going to sell this thing."

If Fortune Management can catch them at midlife crisis, or even when they dip down into aging, we can still turn it around and bring them back up the mountain. We can still help them to help themselves. But it only gets uglier from there: as they get further into aging, now everything is aging—not just the doctor and his or her energy level but the team is aging, the patient base is aging, the facility is aging, and the equipment is outdated.

Now they've got a real problem because it's affecting the valuation of their business. If they ignore the issue, then they go into the next phase—institutionalization. This phase for a dental practice is, again, no different than it is for human beings who cannot support themselves on their own. They're on artificial respiration, so to speak. For a dental practice that means the business is no longer profitable and is being kept alive by artificial means, like tapping into retirement accounts or borrowing money from banks. These practices are what we've referred to previously as teardown practices.

At that point, with a teardown practice, common thinking holds that there are only two places it can go: It gets closed down and be worth nothing (death) or it is sold for pennies on the dollar. But these aren't the only options available. The good news for a later-career dentist with a teardown practice, even if the practice is well along the aging process or even in the institutionalization stage, is that it can be salvaged by being paired with another of our clients—an earlier-career doctor whose practice is in the zone of maximization.

How does that work? Those late-career doctors, even if they've reached the teardown phase, often retain two very valuable assets: their reputation and their patient base. That sets the stage for us being able to take someone who is beyond midlife crisis and into aging and even institutionalization and match them with a younger practice in the teenage, young adult, or maturity stage.

For doctors at the top of their game, those currently in the zone of maximization, our question is, Why not bring in another doctor's practice—where that doctor has a great reputation and loyal patient base but whose practice is aging—and create economies of scale so your business can experience another arc of growth?

Limiting Beliefs

Two types of thinking limit doctors' ability to consider this paradigm shift. Neither involves how they run their practices but rather how they think about their finances.

The first limiting belief is thinking they know everything about the financial side of things. There are some dentists who think that because they've got great clinical skills, they're also financial wizards. Yet no matter how much they think they know about finances, they're trained to practice dentistry; they haven't studied business, investing, or entrepreneurship. Because they think they know everything, many of these folks get into pretty sad shape. Whatever they think is working works, until it doesn't, and then they're really behind the eight ball.

The other limiting belief is thinking they don't have enough critical mass in their portfolio. In other words, they think they don't have enough money or know-how to play the game. They think, "I really don't know much about finances. I'd rather do nothing. I'd rather not have a plan in place because it's something I don't understand and it makes me uncomfortable. I just don't want to play the game."

We know where that mindset ends up. When doctors get on the back side of that bell curve, they start hearing voices, whether from practice brokers or themselves: "What could have been one of the greatest assets in my portfolio is now not worth much."

We've heard many doctors say, "I'm just going to close it down and walk away." Or, "I'm just going to sell the old equipment or donate the old equipment to charity and take the tax write-off."

This can be a self-fulfilling prophecy that results in the continued erosion of their practice, and it starts with some really ugly limiting beliefs about what their practice is worth if it's put in the right hands. Those are the folks we need to do an intervention with right away because it's not too late to save them. We can come in and not radically change the practice, but maybe make a five-, ten-, or fifteen-degree turn that will double, triple, or quadruple their results.

The issue is not getting more patients in the chair or getting more revenue; it's not a tax issue or a debt issue. The issue is never what they think it is. Almost always, it's an eight-inch issue, which is the distance between a person's right and left ears. When we open their eyes to alternative solutions, that's when the healing begins. That's when everything becomes possible again. They stop dealing with what is and start dealing with what could be and turning that into a reality.

The number one thing an entrepreneur has to do is protect his or her confidence. We find that when clients are in bad shape personally, professionally, and financially, often the number one cause is that they've lost confidence. We help them restore the confidence they need to get past their limited thinking.

Life Cycle of Your Career

There are two life cycles for every dentist: the life cycle of their asset—the brick-and-mortar practice that they own, which we've been discussing—and the life cycle of their career. That's a different matter from their asset. We're asking readers to be honest about the condition of their practice and about where they see themselves in the life cycle of their career.

The latter question typically gets later-career dentists to consider how they want to go out—whether they want to put themselves in a new environment where they can enjoy maybe an additional five years on the back end of their career, or whether they just really feel like they're done.

If we can come in during the midlife phase and establish a strong culture, structure, and strategy, we can turn things around for the midlife crisis doctor. We can help those doctors be self-sufficient again. But when a practice reaches the aging, institutionalized, or even near-death phases, the path forward is to be acquired by another practice so the dentists can maximize their earn-outs. Dentists who are in teardown mode have a practice worth pennies on the dollar. But often we can take that same asset and move it under the roof of a successful Fortune-managed office, creating much higher earn-out valuations in a tax-deferred manner.

Helping Practices on the Decline

There aren't many others in this industry doing these kinds of deals. For us, it's about helping the profession of dentistry as a whole—not just helping the most successful practices, which we do every day, but helping to advance this profession and caring about doctors on a human level. That means helping practices that are declining. We've come in and changed people's lives, and we view it as a calling. It's not the most lucrative part of Fortune or Sequoia, but it's the most meaningful.

To be candid, some folks in the dental community don't have the skill set or desire to help practices in the midlife, aging, or institutionalization stages. Teardown practices aren't desirable listings for practice brokers, who are understandably reluctant to sign a six-month leasing agreement for a business that's tough to market. It's the equivalent of a realtor taking a listing for a beat-up house that's in a bad area.

We can take that same asset and boost its worth to 75 percent of annual collections and improve on that by transferring the old patient base to a new environment. We then put that newly merged practice on steroids. Moving an existing patient base into a new practice has the power to transform a practice from institutionalization to viable retirement asset.

Remember that this conversation about life cycle is for doctors at the beginning, middle, and end of the bell curve. No matter where your practice is in the life cycle, wherever we find a client or a client finds us, we can create a success story. If you're at the beginning, we'll show you how to grow, build, and acquire. If you're in the maturity phase, we'll show you how to experience another arc of growth. If you're on the back side of the curve, it's about either bringing you back fully to the zone of maximization or giving you a best-case scenario liquidity event so you can go out on top.

At some point, typically later in the life cycle of a dental practice, a dentist wants to cash out. Proper preparation for selling a practice is half the battle, one we'll cover next.

Chapter 5

HOW TO PREPARE A
PRACTICE FOR SALE

There comes a time in every dentist's career that calls for serious consideration of selling the practice. If you are a mid- to late-career dentist, you might conclude, for a variety of reasons, that you no longer want to own your practice. Perhaps you want to liquefy your assets into your investment portfolio, or you have simply decided that it's time to retire.

Regardless of what has brought you to this crossroads in your career, you have a variety of options to help you reach this goal. Which of these strategic approaches is best for you, however, really depends on the timeline you have mapped out and how that fits into your life plan. Remember, you must always begin with the end in mind.

There are alternatives to selling your practice with a conventional, cash walkaway sale. The cash walkaway sale is basically the process of putting the practice up for sale, finding a buyer, and getting paid a negotiated price for it. With this method, the owner stays on for a very short transitional period, usually no more than six months from the date of sale, but ultimately walks away from the practice entirely.

At that point, the dentist no longer has a place to work, which means the dentist no longer has a place where he or she can trade time for dollars. And in most cases, the selling dentist also forfeits access to a business entity for tax purposes. This method of selling is the most conventional, but it isn't your only option.

You can also exit your practice through transition planning. With this method, you can bring in the next-generation dentist, who ultimately will buy the practice over an extended period. While the end result is the same as the cash walkaway sale, the difference is that as the initial owner you may stay on for a predetermined time and possibly work as an associate to the new owner. You may even do this in phases so that you don't sell 100 percent of the practice right away, but maybe just one-third or half at a time.

A third option for exiting your practice is to be acquired by another existing practice. This gives you the option to stay on as an associate dentist. You may even collaborate on an earn-out program—a process that we'll discuss in chapter 10, "How to Finance the Purchase or Sale of a Practice"—which essentially sets up the dentist to earn out of his or her practice over three to five years.

Now, the benefits of all three exit options really depend on your life plan as well as your current health and financial situation. In all cases, though, if we are going to prepare for a sale and make a series of effective decisions to prepare your practice for any of these options, we must begin with the end in mind. Once you know your short- and long-term goals and take your financial situation into consideration, you can decide which exit option is best for you. Each method requires different preparation.

In a cash walkaway sale of the practice, potential buyers and lenders are going to be looking at certain aspects of the business:

- Condition of the facility

- Quality of the lease
- Condition of the equipment
- Condition of the patient base (age, health, demographics, etc.)
- Systems and processes in place
- The team
- Top-line volume annual lead
- Bottom-line profitability
- Standard of care and hygiene
- Recare efficiency

There are more-detailed lists of what will be scrutinized, depending on the type of practice, but these comprise a basic checklist of items that should be in sound working order so that you can get the maximum valuation for your practice.

If you choose to pursue the second option, which would be a longer period during which a doctor would want to transition into working with the new doctor, you will not necessarily focus on preparing for the initial sale, but on how the practice can accommodate a second doctor. The best way to begin this is by interviewing younger doctors and letting them know that the ultimate outcome of the relationship would be for them to be the owner.

In other words, the older doctor transitioning would want to start with a conversation about hiring not an associate, but a future partner and ultimately the owner of the business. You would still need to factor in how the practice could accommodate salaries for both doctors, as well as who would make decisions and what the process of making major decisions for the practice would look like. A great deal of planning must take place for this to be successful.

The level of nuanced preparation that needs to take place even when you are planning on staying on for an extended period can be daunting. The most obvious requirement, and perhaps the most important in preparing for this scenario, is to find a younger doctor who shares your goals and has the energy to take on the management, leadership, or day-to-day dentistry tasks that you no longer want to handle.

There must also be a growth plan for the practice. A common mistake that dentists make is to bring on an associate without having a growth plan in place, which means that they are now supporting two doctors' incomes with the same amount of revenue that was previously supporting one salary. This, obviously, curtails profitability. To avoid this situation, you must decide with the younger doctor whether you will grow through enhanced marketing, through more insurance plans, or through mergers and acquisitions; there are a lot of conversations to be had there.

The third option for exiting the practice, which is to have it acquired by another existing practice, has a preparation process similar to that of the cash walkaway sale to maximize valuation. However, as with the second option, you must also work out the details of how much of the practice will be sold and when, what your role will be as you earn out, and whether you are still taking on leadership responsibilities. Or perhaps you will decide to sell it entirely and have the practice fully acquired by another existing practice.

The acquisition can proceed in a couple of different ways. Certainly, the conventional way is for the buyer to review the facility, lease, and equipment, and determine if it is a teardown practice. Essentially, this means that its only intrinsic value is the doctor's reputation and the patient base. This kind of scenario requires a different preparation strategy to maximize your liquidity event and earn-out.

Another way this third option can play out is in the case of a superior facility with great equipment and sound infrastructure; in such a situation, we could also be looking for a reverse merger—another practice reverse merges into that existing location.

Regardless of which option you choose, maximizing your outcome requires a compelling story about the quality of that business. When it comes to the sale of any business, as we have said before, three things make the difference between just doing an asset sale and selling a company that has intrinsic value and getting top dollar for it: great culture, structure, and strategy. Without these, you cannot expect to net full price for the sale—it would not be a sound decision for the buyer, and lenders most likely won't finance the purchase.

These are only some of the issues you must explore before you begin the process of selling, and this is why we cannot stress enough the value of bringing in experts who will help you begin with the end in mind. How you prepare for your exit or your transition cannot be determined until you are clear on why you are doing it and how it affects your life as the owner-doctor.

* * *

When working with doctors who want to sell, retire, or transition, we frequently find ourselves asking questions that dig far below the surface so that we can find out why the doctor has come to this juncture at this point in their career. Have they made this decision solely based on their age? Their financial situation? Maybe they are struggling, or perhaps they simply desire a different lifestyle. We work to reveal those reasons and then work backwards to arrive at the desired outcome and the best process to achieve it.

As it comes down to preparing your practice for sale, regardless of your goal and the method you choose for pursuing it, you need to have some things in your toolkit to be successful: time and the right team.

We often see doctors encounter tragedy because they start this process two weeks prior to selling, when they should have brought us in to begin preplanning five to ten years ago. And we mention the "right team" because the reality is that many individuals and companies out there call themselves transition specialists or coaches, but they aren't equipped to provide the expert guidance to prepare a practice for sale to maximize the valuation and the outcome.

Another significant contribution that the right team will make as you prepare your practice for sale is to help you make logical decisions and avoid emotional ones. If a doctor called us today and stated that she had thought it over and concluded that the best option for her was to find a broker and do a cash walkaway sale, we would ask, "How do you know that you're right?"

As the selling doctor, you may think you know what's right for you. But anytime you arrive at a decision, it is best to go deeper and ask how you know you are right. How do you know that taking this path is the right choice for you? When looking at all the components to any one decision logically, you can retrace your steps to identify how you know that you are right. But when you arrive at a conclusion based on emotion, you often cannot identify, logically, why you are so sure.

* * *

There's no way to prepare for the sale of your asset if you haven't first considered how it fits into your life plan, financial plan, and career plan. These three questions have everything to do with how we prepare.

Determining which of the three exiting options is best for you depends on various criteria, and each option will yield different benefits for you depending on your lifestyle, financial needs, and life plan. If an older doctor no longer feels the need to hold a handpiece, then the best option is a straightforward acquisition. It is unlikely that this doctor would benefit from a long-term transition plan with a younger doctor. But if a doctor still loves the trade and enjoys treating patients—and simply no longer wants to be an owner—then the longer transitional period is likely the best option.

The most important thing to remember when preparing for a sale is that no two deals are the same, and no two transitions look alike. When working with a client preparing for a sale, we ask questions about the value of the practice, the desire to get the liquidity event out of the sale, the client's financial planning, their long-term goals, and much more. We are fully aware of the doctor's life and that of the practice before we even begin to guide them toward whichever option is best.

Chapter 6

DETERMINING THE VALUE OF THE PRACTICE YOU SEEK TO BUY OR SELL

We evaluate the practice from many different dimensions, then triangulate all the observations to arrive at its true value.

As with selling a home, car, or any other asset, when it comes to buying or selling a dental practice, the market determines the price— that is, it is worth what someone is willing to pay for it. But price isn't everything; it is only one aspect of the value of a practice, albeit a significant factor.

Other factors in determining the value of a practice include the top-line annual collections and what a lender will finance on the asset. The national average of what conventional underwriters and lenders today are willing to lend is 70 to 80 percent. In other words, if a dental business earns $1 million a year, odds are that we can go out and secure 100 percent financing on up to $700,000 to $800,000. Though less common, it is sometimes possible to secure financing for up to 90 percent of a practice's value.

Another way we view evaluation is in multiples of bottom-line earnings, often known in business transactions as EBITDA, which measures a company's operating performance. Typically, practices can go for anywhere between two and three times the bottom-line EBITDA, averaging about two and a half times. While useful, this number, too, is dependent upon the market.

It is important to note that across the country, local economies are not all the same. Some are buyers' markets; others are sellers' markets. These trends usually go in cycles, but if you're buying or selling you cannot necessarily wait for market trends to change. You may not be able to plan around market trends, but you do want to be aware of them because they are a significant factor in determining the value of a practice.

Several additional factors must be taken into account when evaluating the value of a practice. Many of the items discussed in chapter 5 that go into preparing a practice for sale are also key components of value:

- Condition of the facility
- Quality of the lease
- Condition of the equipment
- Condition of the patient base (age, health, demographics, etc.)
- Systems and processes in place
- The team
- Top-line volume annual lead
- Bottom-line profitability
- Standard of care and hygiene
- Recare efficiency

Still, determining the value of a practice is not as straightforward as preparing one for sale, despite the overlap in factors for consideration. For instance, a good-quality lease in place can be seen as an asset as well as a liability, as it could enhance the gross rent multiplier. Higher profitability will also enhance the gross multiplier for evaluation. We must also take into account the buyer's and the seller's attitudes toward the maximum or minimum sale price.

It is important to note that it is rare to find someone willing to sell a mature practice. This is another area where you really need an expert to review all the factors for a fair evaluation. Often we find that a practice for sale is experiencing wide swings, and many are experiencing decline. Prior to selling, many doctors have neglected recare or practice renewal, so that the bottom line may be higher, but maintaining the practice will cost the purchasing doctor later on.

Conversely, the doctor may have invested in pumping up the practice to show a higher bottom line and net greater market value for the practice, yet the growth is not sustainable over the long term. The purchasing doctor may have no idea what he or she is actually getting into with that practice.

A seasoned professional will be able to discover the story behind the numbers and evaluate the practice comparatively. Let's look at a scenario of Practice A versus Practice B. Both practices show top-line collections of $1 million, but that does not mean that both practices should be valued equally at $1 million.

Practice A may have $1 million that drives $500,000 to the bottom line, which is far above industry average for profitability. However, going into the practice for an in-depth evaluation, we may discover large amounts of deferred maintenance needed on the equipment and other major necessary upgrades. We may also find that the lease is up for renewal in the next one to two years. The patient base may also be aging so that much of the dentistry has already been completed and the future will not see the same bottom-line results. If the dentist has focused on the bottom line and has not invested in constant renewal of the practice, that makes a huge difference for the buying dentist.

Industry average is to pay about 80 to 90 percent of the value, but to do so on a practice such as Practice A can be problematic. The new dentist will be entering that practice with the whole of that loan to repay, and on top of it will face patient turnover as well as team turnover, not to mention the costs of rebranding and marketing efforts. In addition to these costs, the purchasing dentist will potentially have to put hundreds of thousands of dollars into the renewal of the facility and the equipment. That $500,000 in bottom-line profit may no longer seem so attractive.

In comparison, let's evaluate Practice B. This practice may be driving only 20 percent to the bottom line compared to Practice A's 50 percent, but that's because Practice B has recently invested in equipment and other upgrades that have yet to contribute to profitability. It may also be that the selling dentist is investing in marketing and renewal efforts, which will reduce the amount of time and money the new dentist will have to spend in those areas, but those efforts will have a long-term positive impact.

These are the nuances that a skilled professional can help you evaluate before making a decision to buy and at how much. Keep in mind, as we covered in chapter 2, that no two deals are the same. It is impossible for anyone to render an opinion on the value of a practice without a specific, in-depth evaluation.

None of this is to imply that a practice must be perfect for a doctor to buy or sell it. There is value in the purchase or sale of nearly every type of practice, and what that value is depends on your goal. For instance, some doctors may find themselves in the situation of needing to sell a teardown practice, which may be tied to a horrible lease, relying on poor equipment, with a health-challenged patient base, an aging doctor, and dwindling profitability. This practice is at the institutionalization stage, where the doctor is not even making any money.

In this situation, we'd have to take an in-depth look at all the possibilities and have an important conversation with the selling doctor. The reality is that if he tries to do a cash walkaway sale, the evaluation is going to be forty or fifty cents on the top-line dollar.

On the other hand, if we can match the doctor with the right acquisition partner, we can potentially bring that up to seventy-five cents on the dollar. Again, when determining the value of the practice, it is essential to work with a team of professionals who know what they're doing. They can help you achieve your goal of selling while ensuring greater profit simply by adjusting your exit strategy.

Cash flow is another important factor to consider when determining the value of a practice that you are buying or selling. If you are looking for a younger doctor to either buy your practice or slowly begin partnering in it, then you must keep in mind that cash flow is very important. A new doctor who is going out and borrowing the money to purchase the practice will be coming in with a hefty loan to repay. We often have to caution sellers here because while they obviously want the practice to be worth more, the reality is that if the price is too high, the young doctor cannot prove that he or she will be able to service the debt. That means that a bank will not lend for your practice, which greatly limits potential buyers.

Another aspect to consider is whether you have existing debt on the practice. That also will make a big difference on the bottom line for potential lenders. An older doctor may have just bought a $150,000 piece of equipment that is now a lease payment against the business, and while that may increase profit down the line, it will also limit cash flow.

A final word of caution to dentists about determining the value of a practice: If you are looking to buy, you are likely to encounter doctors who have a strong emotional attachment to their practices. They know that there is a certain number that they need in order to retire or that they need out of the liquidity event, and that is what they are focused on, regardless of the truth about the actual worth of their asset. In such cases, the selling doctor has thrown logic completely out the door, and it is up to you, the buyer, to avoid making an emotional decision in buying that practice. Paying too much for a practice can be dangerous, especially if you are a young doctor taking out a loan to do so.

Determining the value of any practice, whether you buying or selling, involves a complicated evaluation process that takes multiple factors into consideration. Again, it is important to keep in mind that no two practices are the same, and no two deals are the same. Each transaction, to maximize its full potential and achieve your end goal, requires a unique evaluation conducted by skilled professionals.

Chapter 7

MAKING THE DEAL WORK
FOR BOTH SIDES

The M&A process we've developed works for both buyer and seller, including sellers who have teardown practices.

From the buyer's side, it's a very basic premise: The buyer wants to drive more revenue through the same fixed overhead. The buyer finds a practice down the street and merges it with his or her existing practice. There are no loans required, and the buyer pays only for the patients who transfer over. By paying the selling doctor either on an earn-out basis or with bank financing, 40–50 percent of every dollar from that new practice will drop right to the bottom line.

So, by buying a million-dollar practice and merging it into an existing facility, the new owner could conservatively bring $400,000–$500,000 to the bottom line. This can be accomplished by bank financing, seller financing, and many times a hybrid of the two. There is little or no risk with an earn-out, and strategic risk is only present when bank financing is necessary. (We'll talk more about financing in chapter 10, "*How to Finance the Purchase or Sale of a Practice.*")

It's pretty straightforward for the buying doctor to see why it makes sense. On the seller's side, though, the argument is a bit more complicated. Often sellers are being counseled by their attorney, accountant, or spouse to avoid a merger: "Hey, you've got to do a cash walkaway deal. You don't want to take the risk."

We say, what risk? If you relocate to a new, beautiful facility and treat the patients you've been treating for the last twenty, thirty, or forty years, where's the risk? Your patients will remain with you, except now you will be treating them in a superior facility with updated equipment, better systems and patient reactivation, and higher reimbursements from insurance carriers. How is that any risk?

What we do is lower the risk for each party—creating a lot more wealth for both parties. Late-career dentists who heed those naysayers pushing them toward a cash walkaway sale are often making a very costly decision. For the doctor selling, a cash walkaway sale does not maximize the sale opportunity—neither in the amount of money made nor in the potential psychological benefits of handing off the business responsibilities while continuing to do what they love.

M&A versus Cash Walkaway

Today, there are about five thousand teardown dental practices in the US. The only things of intrinsic value they retain are the patient base and presumably the doctor's reputation in the community.

It's important to understand that teardowns are the least favorite practices for brokers to sell because they lack profitability, an attractive location or facility, and a favorable lease. They're also highly unappealing to young dentists seeking practices to purchase. Because they're the least attractive for a broker to sell, resale prices are extremely low. Consequently, our approach to making the deal work for both sides creates a huge win for sellers compared to a cash walkaway option.

Opting for an M&A over a cash walkaway sale yields two significant benefits for the selling doctor: First, the doctor has the chance to make far more money in the long run because taxes are deferred. Second, it provides the many psychological benefits of no longer having to run a business. Selling doctors can practice on their patients with no management requirements.

Many doctors feel burned out. "I love the dentistry I'm doing; I just hate the business part of it," many say. That's really why we do this work: We want those doctors to enjoy the freedom of concentrating on what they love to do. If they can cash out of the business side at an optimal time—three, four, or five years before they're ready to slow down or stop holding a handpiece—then they're free from the responsibility of running the business while still generating a steady income.

Through an M&A, dentists selling their practices earn a lot more money in the long run than a cash walkaway sale would produce. With the latter, the seller pays all the capital gains tax in one year and dissolves his or her professional corporation. An M&A, on the other hand, allows taxes to be deferred and the doctor to retain a professional corporation structure.

In chapter 11 we'll talk about turbocharging your newly merged practice. That applies to both sides: We're turbocharging it for both buyer and seller. For the late-career doctor who's selling, it's about maximizing the practice's valuation in that doctor's final years.

Example M&A: $800,000 Buyer and $500,000 Seller

We know that the average general practitioner generates around $800,000 in top-line annual collections. Let's sketch out merging an $800,000 practice with a teardown practice candidate that's generating $500,000.

Going into one of these M&As, it's important to understand the condition of both sides in terms of each doctor's pretax income. Our buyer, who collects $800,000 top-line, has an overhead of 72 percent. That leaves pretax earnings of about $225,000.

There's a good possibility that the seller—the doctor running the $500,000 practice—is only seeing a 10–20 percent profit, and could actually be losing money to keep the practice alive. You read in chapter 4 about the life cycle of a business. We know that aging and institutionalization happen at the end of the life cycle, and institutionalization is the last step before death, whether it's a human being or a business that happens to be a dental practice.

We know it won't be difficult to convince the acquiring dentist that it will work; if the buyer can take that $500,000 in revenue and the selling doctor's good reputation and move them under that $800,000 roof, he or she has created a $1.3 million practice. None of the fixed costs—rent, or any debt financing that might be in place on the $800,000 practice—change. Only some of the variable costs change, and not by much.

For the buyer, there's huge upside. Of that $500,000, about 60 percent of it, or $300,000, is likely to drop to the buyer's bottom line. So what have we done? We have, with a few pen strokes and a little bit of work in the M&A process, changed the income level of our buyer from $225,000 to more like half a million.

There are many reasons why it should be a win for our seller, too. Once the practices merge, the seller has immediately eliminated all previous overhead costs. The seller gets to do what he or she really loves, and earn 30 percent of restorative collections as real income.

At the same time, the seller will be entitled to an earn-out percentage from the buyer. It can be based on anywhere from one to five years, with a percentage ranging from 50 to 80 percent of annualized collections over that period.

In many cases, selling doctors will still be able to fund their current retirement plan. They've eliminated overhead. They'll be able to create a liquidity event out of their asset in a tax-deferred manner, over a series of tax years.

We often talk in seminars about "common thinking." This is the path most people follow, and it controls very little of the wealth in this country. People assume common thinking is the safe strategy. Our experience, however, is that the safe strategy is sometimes riskier than the opportunities that create a lot more wealth. It's really uncommon thinking that controls most of the wealth in this country. And that's what we want our readers to see: we want them to consider uncommon thinking.

When's the Right Time for an M&A Deal?

It's vital to follow a process to prepare for this kind of deal. When is the right time for the selling doctor? Multiple factors affect the timing.

One important factor is whether there are lease obligations on the practice. If a few years remain on the lease, that's a factor we have to mitigate. The best scenario is that the lease is up for renewal within the next twelve months. Another factor is whether the business has any long-term debt or secured liens. There's also the question of whether the selling doctor is ready to relinquish primary control of the practice. It's a difficult but important question: Is that doctor willing and able to effectively hand off the practice to another doctor, and not have the same control or authority?

While some control will necessarily have to be given up, remember that this process allows the selling doctor to put his or her name on the door of the newly merged practice. It's not a retirement. Instead, the message to patients should be that we're merging into a group practice to improve the patient experience and raise the standard of care.

There's a proven process to identifying and pursuing practices that are good candidates for acquisition. We'll cover that next chapter.

Chapter 8

HOW TO BE AN OPPORTUNISTIC BUYER

An opportunistic buyer is always asking how to bring in another great doctor and another great patient base. How can we take better advantage of economies of scale? An opportunistic buyer looks for solo practitioners who aren't sold on the idea of remaining solo.

This mindset relates to trends in dentistry. As we wrote in the introduction, the days of the single practitioner—working four days a week, shouldering the entire burden of staff expenses, new technology investment, and facility costs—are disappearing.

There will always be boutique practice owners who choose to do it that way, of course. They prefer to do it all themselves, and we understand that, but it is not the most effective economic model and it is no way to compete in an era of corporate dentistry.

Letters and Warmer Leads

Opportunistic buyers follow a two-step process to get deals on the table: letters and warmer leads. We start by sending a letter to every practice in which at least 75–80 percent of the patients would be willing to travel to your office. The boundaries obviously depend on the area: In major metropolitan cities, that might be a ten-square-

DATE

Dear Colleague,

I hope this letter finds you and your practice doing well. I am writing to you because I am looking to expand my practice either through a merger or a transitional partnership.

My practice in _____ has been open since _____. I am fortunate to work with a highly motivated team of professional and friendly staff. We will be moving into a brand new facility by the end of the year with our continued emphasis on high tech/high touch dentistry: digital radiography, Cerec Omnicam, several dental laser frequencies for both hard and soft tissues, etc.

If you are considering a transition in your practice, whether it's having more time at home with your family, or having a partner to help take on the administrative portion of your business, or looking to retire in the near future and want to provide your patients with a more gentle transition, I would be interested in talking with you. Some of the benefits of this type of partnership or transition are not having to be on call every week and avoiding broker fees.

Cash Buy Out of $800K Annual Practice Appraised at 70%
$56,000.00
$240,000.00
$504,000.00
☐ brokerage fees (10%) ☐ Pre-Tax Final Take Home ☐ Apraisal loss

Fortune 3 Year Buy Out of $800K Annual Practice Appraised at 75%
$150,000.00 $50,000.00
$400,000.00
☐ Profit from Selling Shell/Equipment ☐ Base Take Home ☐ Apraisal loss

There are many types of partnerships and transitions and it is important to find one that will benefit all parties involved, our patients, our staff, and our practices. If you are interested, please contact me at _____ or _____. Any discussions on this topic will be held in strictest confidence.

Sincerely,

block area; in Wyoming, it might be a hundred square miles. In Rockland County, New York, for example, Nyack and Tarrytown are three miles apart, but nobody crosses the Tappan Zee Bridge to visit the dentist. The letter describes your offer and what's special about the way you do business.

The second step is pursuing warmer leads. Veteran dentists typically know the other dentists in the community, so we get the word out to them that you are looking for acquisition candidates. When you are buying, you want the world to know. You want your staff to know. You want suppliers and practice brokers to know. Practice brokers are your friends when you're buying, because the seller pays the commission, so you want as many brokers as possible looking for potential practices to buy.

Once you have someone on the phone, you can ask, "Hey, Joe. Hey, Susie. Have you done any thinking about your transition or your exit strategy? I've got some ideas for a way we can do something better together than we can apart. Are you free for coffee or lunch next week?" Then we prepare you for that meeting.

Success Builds on Success

We tell a story in live seminars about a young dentist Fortune Management took on seven years ago. At the time, this doctor was running a small, $300,000 practice in a three-chair facility he had bought from a seventy-eight-year-old retiring dentist. It was not a good facility, and this young dentist had very limited growth opportunities.

But there were other opportunities, and we helped him figure out what they were. He was in a professional building centrally located in a major metropolitan area, and there were eighty other dentists in the same building. If we could find an older practitioner who was looking for an exit strategy and had a more suitable facility, we could do a reverse merger, taking our $300,000-a-year practice and reverse merging it into a $500,000-a-year practice with five chairs. If we could find that kind of doctor to partner with on an M&A, we would create three wins: an $800,000 practice, growth opportunities for the younger doctor, and an attractive exit strategy for the older doctor.

We did find a suitable partner—an older doctor in the same building who was looking for an exit strategy—but he didn't end up retiring right away. He stayed with that practice for another five years.

After that first M&A, we identified another late-career dentist in the same building, whose practice was earning about $300,000–$400,000 a year, and we brought him under the same roof. We moved him up four floors into this facility, and at the same time we did a complete facility remodel. When we were done with the acquisition and remodel, we now had a $1.5 million practice.

We didn't stop there. We started focusing on organic growth through economies of scale, because now we had a group practice with three doctors. We expanded to a $2.5 million practice by using the turbocharging strategies we'll talk about in chapter 11, and by taking advantage of the synergy the two mergers had created.

We didn't stop there. Now the practice was outgrowing the space, so we identified a $1.5 million practice owned by a dentist who was sixty years old and still at the peak of his career. That merger gave us the ability to move into a brand-new, state-of-the-art, twelve-chair facility, creating what is now a $4 million-a-year practice. Our clients also own the real estate where the practice sits.

Their organic growth continues. The expanded facility has allowed us to bring multiple specialties under one roof, which, as we know, is a key part of the future of dentistry.

Ultimately, we grew a $300,000 single practitioner into a $4 million group practice, which will soon be a $5–$6 million practice because the owners are continuing to leverage turbocharging strategies and economies of scale.

The amazing thing about this success story is that all those opportunities were found right inside the same building.

What we did along the way—taking that $300,000 practice through three M&As and organically expanding it into what is now a twelve-chair, $4 million and growing practice—has improved many people's lives. The deals benefited all three doctors whose practices

were acquired. We helped them create compelling financial strategies for their liquidity event, and two of the three doctors are still
working as associates today. We also improved the lives of thousands
of patients, who now enjoy care in the finest dental facility in that
city.

Chapter 9

EXITING YOUR PRACTICE ON YOUR OWN TERMS

There are many different scenarios for exiting. We've spent years developing creative approaches to this M&A process so that doctors who have dedicated careers to their patients and profession can exit on their own terms—i.e., in a way that benefits them both financially and psychologically.

To exit your practice on your own terms, you must plan ahead. It's critical to start thinking about these things long before you're actually ready to exit. Preparation allows you to do it your way.

Money isn't the only consideration in planning an exit strategy. Many late-career doctors are tied up in what they do and the relationships with their staffs and the patients who love them. These doctors don't necessarily want to withdraw from their business. They want to work less, but they aren't ready to put down the handpiece. They want to continue to practice, but without the stress—to take their chips off the table and just enjoy their patients and their life.

Working Back as an Associate

One of the most popular scenarios for exiting is selling the asset and working back as an associate. Typically the buying doctor brings on a minority partner who wants to continue practicing dentistry as an associate for a number of years. One doctor merges into another doctor's practice. The selling doctor continues to work on his or her own patients as an associate, ultimately transitioning those patients over to the buying doctor.

We have specific compensation formulas for the selling doctor who works back as an associate. The formula always reflects the doctor's particular skills and preferences.

This is all written into the operating partnership agreement—the most important document in a successful merger. The devil is the details, and the better crafted the partnership agreement, the fewer problems and disagreements arise.

Over the years, we've seen many selling doctors who have been acquired and merged who expected to stay on as an associate for six months or a year. But they ended up loving the situation so much that they stayed on for five years. Those extra years made the sale even more attractive, because it meant additional revenue as an associate, far beyond the liquidity event.

When doctors reach their fifties and sixties, continuing to practice dentistry becomes a physical challenge. Dentistry is both a physical and a mental grind. We're seeing a lot of doctors who've been working four and a half or five days a week for thirty years. They're tired. But when we give them permission to cut back to three, two and a half, or two days a week, then their neck, their back, their legs, and their minds all get refreshed.

At that point, many of them think, "Hey, if I could do this two or three days a week, I don't want to retire." By working back as an associate, these doctors can extend their careers while enhancing both their finances and their enjoyment of life.

When one doctor joins another doctor's practice as an associate, the working relationship between the partnering doctors varies from merger to merger. Sometimes, the selling doctor can check out of the business side of things because the younger, buying doctor has all the skills to run that business. In that scenario, the older doctor can simply enjoy his or her patients, staff, and what's left of his or her career.

Other times, the older doctor takes on a mentor role because the younger doctor isn't quite ready to be in the number one chair. Even though the younger doctor might own a majority of the practice, because that doctor is not yet ready to execute it flawlessly, the older doctor assumes some of the leadership responsibilities.

Done Holding a Handpiece—Going Fishing

Doctors who don't want to work anymore and just want to go fishing or golfing can leave on their own terms, too. But even though that's what their goal is, we want those doctors to understand that does not mean they must do a cash walkaway sale.

They can still be acquired and merged. That generally requires only three to six months. Investing that additional three to six months on the trailing end will make the deal much more attractive for the younger, buying doctor.

Many late-career doctors no longer want to be in the business of dentistry, and they don't have to be. These folks can get out in a way that, again, is beneficial psychologically and financially—without having to do a cash walkaway sale.

The bottom line is, the cash walkaway method—saying, cold turkey, "I'm done as of next Monday"—is a horrible way to exit a practice. It's not good for the patients. It's not good for the team. It's not good for the doctor's reputation. And it's not good for the buyer, who presumably plans to build on the legacy of the seller's practice.

We strongly advise against a cash walkaway sale unless there's an extenuating circumstance, like a major illness or death.

Done Holding a Handpiece—Not Done Holding onto the Asset

There's a huge difference between an asset liquidity event and retirement. One of the things we've seen trending up is doctors exiting their career but not necessarily exiting their investment.

You can leave behind your dental practice but still own the business. Doctors who no longer want to do the physical work of being a dentist do not have to sell the goose that lays the golden eggs. In other words, we can arrange for them to retain ownership of the practice. Whether they hold onto one-third of it or a majority, they become the CEO—or a silent partner, just holding stock in the company.

That structure creates a much more attractive offer for the younger doctor, who now does not need to obtain a loan. The younger doctor would much rather have the older doctor stay on for one-quarter or one-third of the equity in exchange for dividend checks.

An important aspect of our method is coaching doctors to keep their corporations or legal entities active. In many cases, selling doctors can keep their legal entities open for retirement and tax benefits. When it comes to these matters we always advise our clients to consult a CPA and an attorney. There are often lots of ways to continue to keep that entity functioning and be able to accelerate a retirement plan, deduct the appropriate business expenses, and continue to have a more tax-efficient lifestyle.

This process is flexible, and the terms are negotiated based on the relationship between the two doctors. Sometimes if you didn't know better, you would think the doctors were 50/50 business partners when in reality the younger, acquiring doctor owned 100 percent of the practice. It all depends on what the two doctors dream up in terms of how they want to work.

Ego Check

A word of caution to selling doctors: once you've decided that you are going to step back and sell either part or all of your practice—especially if you are going to continue to work back as an associate—you must check your ego at the door.

We have seen many times when a doctor is on board with selling the asset. The doctor wants the liquidity event and still wants to work back as an associate a few days a week. But then he or she wants to act as if they're still the managing partner and owner of the business.

Some doctors want to sell their practice but don't want to be part of the new culture or answer to the new owner, and they become toxic to the practice. It's a classic example of somebody wanting to have their cake and eat it, too. The reality is it's a good way to fail at a transition. The selling doctor must be emotionally ready to give up power, authority, and control of that practice.

* * *

Remember that no two deals are ever the same. How a doctor exits his or her practice always depends on that doctor's lifestyle needs. The exit choices doctors have available depend largely on how much financial preplanning they've done in the five to ten years up to this point. That ramp-up time either makes it either easy or tough for us to do these deals.

Therefore, we advise doctors in the later stages of their careers to reach out to us now. The optimal time to grow a tree was twenty years ago; the next best time is today. When buying a business, the time to think about the exit of that business is right after you buy it. It's never too early to start. The more time doctors give us, the better we can prepare them for the transaction. We can also jump-start their financial planning, setting them up for financial freedom.

Chapter 10

HOW TO FINANCE THE PURCHASE OR SALE OF A PRACTICE

Traditionally, practice deals are done with a bank loan. Instead, we prefer an earn-out agreement over three to five years, putting every patient the selling doctor has into the buying doctor's database. The selling doctor signs an associate contract for the dental work he or she does and we give them, generally, 25 percent of collections over three years or 15 percent over five years.

We like the earn-out model because it aligns the two doctors' interests. They are attached at the hip; it's a true partnership. Both parties are trying to make sure that all patients show up and follow the proper treatment plan. This is different from a cash walkaway sale, which creates no incentive for the selling doctor to ensure a proper transition.

The buyer benefits significantly from an earn-out program. First, an earn-out keeps the exiting doctor's skin in the game, which a cash walkaway sale doesn't. Second, it is a hedge against a major decline in the business revenue. Third, it provides a vehicle to acquire another practice without taking on the risk of a long-term bank loan. No financing is required. There's no debt to report.

All of these build asymmetric risk—low risk with potentially high reward. We highly recommend that our clients always conduct business with asymmetric risk. An earn-out tax-deferred program finances the deal with asymmetric risk, and it does so more creatively than just going to the bank.

For the buyer, the earn-out program directly grows the business: The percentage of collections being paid to the selling doctor reflects increased activity. For the seller, the earn-out program maximizes the tax efficiency of the sale. The selling doctor has the ability, based on personal production and commitment, to obtain up to 15 percent more value on the practice sale than he or she would on a cash walkway sale.

On an average practice collecting $750,000...

3 YEAR EARN OUT - 25% of the Documented Patient Base Collections

Year 1 - Collects $775,000
Selling doctor receives $193,750

Year 2 - Collects $800,000
Selling doctor receives $200,000

Year 3 - Collects $850,000
Selling doctor receives $212,500

Selling doctor receives a total of $606,250 over three years vs $525,000 in one lump sump.

5 YEAR EARN OUT - 15% of the Documented Patient Base Collections

Year 1 - Collects $775,000
Selling doctor receives $116,250

Year 2 - Collects $800,000
Selling doctor receives $120,000

Year 3 - Collects $850,000
Selling doctor receives $127,500

Year 4 - Collects $892,500
Selling doctor receives $133,875

Year 5 - Collects $937,125
Selling doctor receives $140,568

Selling doctor receives a total of $638,193 over five years vs $525,000 in one lump sump.

*Practice numbers illustrate a conservitive growth of 3-5% year over year. In most cases, we apply our methods to achieve a 10-20% growth that maximizes the earnout potential.

The laws governing an earn-out tax-deferred sale vary from state to state. Fortune Management has a group of national alliances in the legal, accounting, and lending fields, as well as with practice brokers, and we are always happy to refer clients to the right people based on their location and the needs of their transition. These professionals all have a role. There's so much synergy in these deals that the M&A process has value to anybody who can help ensure a successful transaction.

* * *

In addition to the earn-out model, hybrid deals—part bank financing and part earn-out—are also becoming more common. Hybrid deals often make sense when the selling doctor has debt. Another scenario hybrid deals solve is when the selling doctor wants the buying doctor to have a little skin in the game, so the buyer borrows some money and we finance the rest with an earn-out.

It's important to note that sometimes we do earn-out deals out of necessity. A major challenge with traditional bank lending is getting money to buy a teardown practice. For example, if we are looking to buy a $500,000 practice that is clearly in decline—bad facility, bad equipment—and the only things left of intrinsic value are the doctor's reputation, the patient base, and a maybe few key employees, the bank is going to say, "What are we lending the $300,000–$400,000 for? This is a bunch of smoke and mirrors. We don't even have collateral that we feel is solid." Sometimes an earn-out is the only way we're going to get it done.

Remember that, ultimately, regardless of whether we're doing an earn-out or a hybrid, this process is not strictly about the math. In the end, it's always an emotional decision that depends on the lifestyle needs of each doctor.

Chapter 11

TURBOCHARGING YOUR NEWLY BOUGHT OR MERGED PRACTICE

When you combine the revenue from two practices into the fixed overhead of one facility, you can really focus on growth. Once the selling doctor's patients are migrated over to the buying doctor's practice, we use various levers to turbocharge the newly merged practice.

Turbocharging strategies give doctors the tools to ensure a healthy bottom line and provide their patients with the best possible clinical care. When Fortune Management takes a dentist and his or her patient base and transplants them into the right setting, that practice grows and succeeds year after year. That's really the beauty of merging an older practice into a younger one, whether through acquisition or partnership: an improved environment for an older doctor and patient base.

Physicians made this kind of migration twenty or thirty years ago. Today, when we can bring two or more dental practices together under one roof and optimize conditions—which means excellence in five areas: facility, technology, team, systems, and culture—all parties win. It's a Class 3 Experience: the doctors, the patients, and the profession of dentistry all win.

Three Levers to Turbocharge

The first lever to turbocharge is profitability, achieved through economies of scale. Any time we can merge two practices and move them under one roof with one set of fixed costs, we're automatically going to increase profitability for both doctors. Whether the acquired doctor is staying on as a partner or not, taking advantage of economies of scale maximizes that doctor's earn out.

The second lever is upping the standard of care. When we bring a patient base into the right environment, we can effectively put it on steroids. Prior to the merger, the selling doctor communicates to patients that the practice is moving into a more modern facility to better serve their needs. When the buying doctor's facility has greater capability and is equipped for more advanced dental procedures, it's possible to provide more comprehensive treatment to the selling doctor's patients.

The patient clearly wins. It's not a difficult sell to migrate them into a better practice that's nearby. For instance, the new facility may be able to do implants. It may be able to treat sleep disorders. It may be able to do more cosmetics. It may be able to do single-appointment crowns and other procedures with techniques like CEREC.

All these technologies maximize the value and productivity of that patient base.

The third lever is recare efficiency. When we merge an older practice with a newer one, improving recare efficiency is low-hanging fruit in the acquisition. When one practice has a better-developed hygiene department, we can focus on high recare efficiency, along with good codiagnosis by the dentist. The average dental practice today has a 30 percent patient reactivation rate. We aim for patient reactivation rates of 50, 60, or 70 percent—and we have some practices over 90.

When we merge a patient base into a practice that has better systems, we can show the whole organization how to work smarter and more efficiently—and have more predictable results. When we transplant any patient base into a practice with a better culture and environment, it improves the patient experience, which directly boosts profitability and productivity.

Three Dimensions of Exponential Growth

We believe the best way to turbocharge your practice is to get coaching from Fortune Management, the leading and largest executive coaching firm for dentists in North America. Fortune has a track record of growing practices by 30–70 percent per year. With our exponential growth methodology we can expand any practice by 30 percent or more, every year, and we have been able to do that for over a quarter century.

Fortune does this by taking advantage of three different strategies to fuel exponential growth: growing the patient base, improving frequency, and earning more per visit.

We accomplish the first strategy, growing the patient base, through marketing and effective referral systems. Marketing is broken up into five areas. Number one is branding/identity. Two is an effective social media program; both of these depend heavily on a great website and consistent social media tactics. Third, we focus on external marketing and new patient acquisition through advertising and referrals. Fourth is internal marketing, which means the spirit of hospitality: How is our practice a remarkable experience for every patient? Number five is better case presentation and enrollment skills—in other words, the power to influence.

The second dimension of exponential growth is frequency. In any business, seeing your customers more often drives growth, so we implement effective recare and reactivation systems.

The third dimension is expanding what we're worth per visit. Entrepreneurial dentists deliver care more cost- and time-efficiently, and there are many ways to do this. Sometimes it's as simple as smart billing practices and mastering the relationship with insurers. Insurance companies are not lining up to say, "We want to pay Dr. X more money for that procedure than we're already paying him." You must be proactively giving insurance networks reasons why they want you in their network and are willing to pay you at the top of the scale.

Beyond using fees and insurance more effectively, there are literally fifty different ways dental practices can earn more per visit. We can expand the menu of services. We can schedule more efficiently to increase productivity. We can bring itinerant specialists into the practice.

Exponential growth means more customers × more frequency × more revenue per visit. We show our doctors how to grow each one of these silos by 10 percent annually, year after year. Collectively, that's a 33 percent improvement in the business: $1.10 \times 1.10 \times 1.10 = 1.33$, or a 133 percent growth factor.

Many times, we've been able to grow practices by 20 percent in each of those silos, which results in a 72 percent bump in the business: $1.20 \times 1.20 \times 1.20 = 1.72$.

This is how Fortune Management has put practices on steroids and grown them for the last quarter century. It's the easy way, not the hard way.

The three dimensions of exponential growth are supported by Fortune's focus on growing practices with better cultures, structures, and strategies. Creating extraordinary practices starts with culture and the maximization of human capital. We make sure that every person in the practice understands the big picture. They understand the concept of open-book management; they understand what it takes to win. Everyone shares the same vision and goals.

When we acquire or merge a practice into another, not only are we improving the bottom line, we're enhancing the environment for the doctors practicing and the patients receiving care. The doctor who is being acquired or merged and is now working in a modernized, more efficient practice may now want to extend his or her career, while the acquiring doctor has increased the size of his or her practice. Both have adopted a more entrepreneurial approach to the business of dentistry and are positioned to create multigenerational wealth for their families.

Chapter 12

CREATING MULTIGENERATIONAL WEALTH IN DENTISTRY

We often sit down with dentists who've been practicing for decades. You look at their tax returns and think, "Wow, this doctor's making a lot of money." Then you look at their net worth and the picture changes. It's absolutely dreadful.

Unlike NFL players, who have an average career of three and a half years, dentists have twenty- to fifty-year careers. There is no reason why dentists cannot create real wealth and, in most cases, multigenerational wealth. They can do it; they just have to make a commitment. Entrepreneurial dentists can not only be financially independent but give their family's next generation the opportunity to be financially independent as well.

Parameters to Wealth Creation.

Before you run, you have to walk. To create multigenerational wealth in dentistry, you need to follow some parameters.

The first parameter involves three basic rules:

1. Live within your means.

2. Save 15 percent or more of your pretax income every year.

3. Protect yourself against lawsuits, creditors, disability, permanent loss of income, and death.

The second parameter is understanding that it's all about liquidity, liquidity, liquidity.

Many doctors have money tied up in their business, real estate, and retirement plans, but they can't write a check for any meaningful amount of money. Liquidity allows you to make intelligent, long-term decisions.

The third parameter is hiring yourself as your own CFO.

To create real wealth, the doctor must be involved in the process. Many doctors who are achieving terrific returns in their practice are not doing the same in their personal finances. But many doctors also spend more time planning family vacations than they do on their finances.

Rather than outsourcing wealth management to a CPA or financial planner, doctors must empower themselves. Being your own CFO is a commitment. You become accountable to yourself, and you cannot let emotion trump logic.

The fourth parameter is not having bad debt.

Good debt—low-cost, tax-deductible fixed debt—is acceptable. Other types of debt are not.

Paychecks and Playchecks

Retirement expert Tom Hegna preaches that all assets should be in one of two classes: paychecks and playchecks.

We help doctors create a portfolio of assets that provides either guaranteed or highly reliable streams of income to replace their paychecks when they stop working. But we don't want all their assets huffing and wheezing trying to produce enough income to replace those paychecks.

We help doctors develop a second level of assets that they can spend and enjoy, or give away, or do whatever they want with. These are playchecks. These assets are not responsible for producing income in retirement; they are free capital and play no role in supporting the doctor's lifestyle.

None of the ways to create true wealth entails holding a handpiece. They are largely passive investments. There are many places to put your money—money market accounts, CDs, IRAs, 401(k)s, stocks, bonds, mutual funds—and most of our clients have some or all of these assets.

At best, however, these are inflation-adjusted holding tanks. In chapter 3, we talked about how real wealth creation—where the money, not the human being, is earning money—comes from owning an operating company, investing in real estate, and financing other deals. All produce earned income over the long term.

Most older doctors start to scale back their chairside dentistry eventually. Some realize they no longer want to be holding a handpiece. Some do so for health reasons. Others figure out that they can earn more money working on the business of dentistry than the practice of dentistry.

We've explained how our system of merging older practices with younger ones often extends the career of the older doctor. Our goal is to have that older doctor continue to produce earned income longer than they would have otherwise, because they don't sell their business at sixty-five—they sell it at seventy or seventy-five or eighty . . . or never. The critical mass in savings they've created does not need to produce income; it can be passed on to the next generation.

Earned Income Beyond Retirement

Most doctors are just draining their assets in their sixties, seventies, and eighties. Yet it's completely possible for these doctors to be adding to their net worth instead of spending it. If, in retirement, you continue to earn more than you spend, that's how you create multigenerational wealth. The only funds you must withdraw are government-mandated required minimum distributions from tax-deferred retirement accounts.

Even if you have a substantial portfolio, when you have no money coming in, it all looks like fixed income over time. Continuing earned income is the way to create real wealth. This means retaining some degree of ownership in your practice—maybe not 100 percent or even 50 percent; maybe it's a minority piece. Having at least some ownership guarantees earned income beyond retirement.

If that earned income from ownership can cover, say, half of your living expenses, then the rest of your assets only need to cover the other half. If ownership income can cover 100 percent of living expenses, then you never have to withdraw any money from the critical mass. You will be a net saver, not a net spender, in retirement, and positioned to pass along lasting wealth to the next generation.

Chapter 13

SHOULD WE CONTINUE
THE CONVERSATION?

Dentists have more options for their transition than ever before. They can sell a practice outright, remain a 10 percent owner, bring in more partners, or anything in between.

For doctors who really know their practices, the transition is a blank canvas. You may be saying, "Well, I know that I want to sell my practice next year," but you don't know what it's worth or who the ideal buyer would be, and you're just going to put a For Sale sign on it. But if you follow that path, you won't be maximizing the asset you've dedicated your career to building.

To optimize your transition, you must become an expert on your practice. The more knowledge you have, the better. The more defined you can make your vision—the better you get to know what you actually have—the more options you have. You must know your practice inside and out, better than anyone else. If you don't know it that way, we can help.

Practice Analysis and Opportunity Assessment

Just as is true of a dental practice, we believe that diagnosing a business without first examining it is malpractice. For us to understand what shape a practice is in now and what a doctor needs for the future, we conduct a practice analysis and an opportunity assessment.

A practice analysis is a way for doctors to get an accurate understanding of where they are right now. They may not know where they want to go, which is fine, but many also don't know where they are at present, and that's not OK. If they're not sure what a good profit and loss statement looks like or what their staff overhead is or what their equipment needs are for the next five years—these are things we need nailed down before we create a transition plan that's going to maximize their payout.

A practice analysis provides objective scrutiny. Most doctors haven't looked at their practice from a different angle, so the analysis often yields results they weren't expecting. For example, some doctors think their practice is maxed out on space—until our analysis finds that they're running at only 70 percent capacity.

It takes a third party to provide that perspective. You return to your same house each day, so you see it in a much different light than does a new guest seeing it for the first time. A different perspective on your practice can reveal growth opportunities.

Our analysis pulls reports from practice management software, but we're also looking beyond the numbers at things you don't find in a spreadsheet. We're interviewing the team and the patients and getting to feel the culture of the practice. We're looking objectively at the systems and strategies that are in place, and we're asking if those serve the practice long term.

Once the practice analysis is complete, then we can focus on what the future could look like—that's the opportunity assessment.

We show doctors a path forward in all the areas currently lacking in their practice. That could determine whether they sell now, because they know their weaknesses up front, or whether they have time to put in a couple of years, improve the practice, and get ten times the return.

Sequoia Private Client Group

In transition planning, it's not enough just to know what the asset is worth. It's vital also to know what position the client is in financially, which will factor into what we have to get out of the asset. We take a holistic approach, knowing that the practice is absolutely connected with the doctor's personal life. One benefits the other.

Along with a practice analysis and opportunity assessment, Fortune Management includes the chance to meet with a Sequoia Private Client Group advisor to analyze the personal finances of the client. Now, all the bases are covered. Instead of considering the silo of the practice on its own, we're looking at the entire view of how a doctor's practice and life are connected.

Don't Wait

You can do something about the things you know need to be done. One of the key messages here is not to wait. When planning a transition, it pays to know what your practice is worth and what the weaknesses are. Give yourself plenty of time to get the outcome you want. If you have time on your side, that gives you more power and leverage.

We find a lot of doctors who continue to put their heads in the sand because they don't want to face the reality of the shape their practice is in. They think, "Oh, I'll just keep my head down and keep working."

They're not taking a proactive approach, looking organically at the practice, and asking, "If I were to step back and hire myself as CEO, what are the things I would change?" Most of the time, they're not asking that question because the answer is a difficult one: they would change themselves.

But that's OK. It's OK if they realize that and get the help they need to improve their leadership skills and business skills. That's where Fortune Management shines: developing the leaders these businesses need to thrive.

Customizable Solutions

We don't have a set agenda. Our consultative sales approach is different in that we determine what's most important to our clients so that we can design a solution that fits their needs. Our solutions are completely customized and unique to match each provider and practice.

It's never appropriate for Fortune, Sequoia, or anyone else in the profession to impose our expectations on the doctor. Nobody can look at a practice from afar and say exactly what that practice needs. It has to be about where that doctor wants to go; it has to be about where you feel you need to be to match your lifestyle needs and career goals.

We come across advisors in our space who treat every client like a nail because the only tool in their toolbox is a hammer. Fortune and Sequoia are different: We offer a wide array of solutions for our providers. Because we have hundreds of different tools in our toolbox, we don't go ripping out drywall to replace the carpet.

In other words, we're not trying to do a complete overhaul. Rather, we keep what doctors have built and take it to the next level. Most providers have been at this a long time. They have a great practice they've built up over decades. They've already molded an amazing vision, and we work within the business model they've created.

Many professionals in our field can't look at a practice and pinpoint the areas that need to be improved, because they don't have the solutions to match. We do. We know there are engines we could turn on and a few leaky faucets we could tweak, to really create the impact our clients want.

Additional Resources

Fortune Management offers the most immersive, postgraduate program available to dentists today. We are the leader in the number of resources provided to dentists.

We get results through a multipronged approach. Every doctor is assigned a front-line executive coach and implementation coach. Every doctor completes a thirty-month accredited training university program with their team (programs are conducted in markets throughout the United States and Canada). And every doctor learns digital dentistry practice management and how to monitor their business with our cloud-based monitoring systems and HR programs—collateral resources you can find on Fortune Management's home page (fortunemgmt.com).

Executive Coaching

Coaching—whether done by a personal trainer, a writing coach, or a business coach—is about two things: identifying where the person is right now and where that person wants to go. Point A to point B.

Doctors are looking for a few key things from an executive coach. They're looking for direction, or a clear road map for getting from point A to point B. They're looking for creativity: Some of it simple, some of it sophisticated—nothing that's too out there or that would put them in jeopardy—but they want some original ideas. And they're also looking for companionship. They want a coach who's not going to give them a self-help book and meet with them a few times, and then say, "Good luck." They want to know there's going to be somebody there every step of the way to take the guesswork out of it.

With the help of an executive coach who brings direction, creativity, and companionship, doctors now have the vision and tools to create a better practice and more lucrative asset.

We have no agenda other than our client's. Being a good coach is taking on that agenda as if it were our own and interacting with that person to get the result that he or she wants. We are in it for the best interest of the client, whether that means growing the practice, selling the practice, or buying more practices.

Great Leaders

When it comes to leadership, we work with our doctors in a number of key areas. One is their belief system. We work on defining the doctor's core beliefs about dentistry, business, and people. What is nonnegotiable? What do they value most that will drive them forward?

In addition to a solid belief system, great leaders have a strong sense of optimism. This does not mean a Pollyanna approach; optimism means that we always have our problem-solver hat on and are focused on solutions.

Great leaders learn to work with a team, and they surround themselves with the very best staff. That means releasing themselves from ego. Doctors who believe that they need to have all the answers become a bottleneck in their own business. Great leaders surround themselves with people who are actually more talented than they are in certain areas. "They fall in love with what they're not," is a quote we particularly like.

Great leaders are strong influencers, which is one level above being a great communicator. The world moves through influence; nothing happens in business unless somebody influences somebody else. No patient accepts treatment unless a quality practice has influenced them.

Integrity and courage are also vital aspects of leadership. Leaders with integrity and courage have the willingness to move forward into this evolving period of dentistry. That doesn't mean they have no fear; it means they have the resolve to move beyond the fear.

Today we probably spend 30 percent of our time in the lab, not just answering questions that clients have now, but anticipating the questions they're going to be asking us six months or a year from now. Just because dental practice transitions have been done one way for decades does not mean they have to continue to be done that way. We believe in challenging the way things have been done to create better ways to serve all parties involved.

We hope in writing this book to affect how this profession practices over the next ten or twenty years. Our overarching goal is to improve the way private practitioners function and evolve in dentistry's new economy.

PRAISE FOR
FORTUNE MANAGEMENT

"Some of our fastest growing practices are the ones working with both Fortune Management and Revenuewell. The practices we see working with Fortune Management are not only ahead of the curve on growth and profitability but have a solid foundation of marketing and customer service in place. Fortune Management's first-time owner program is a terrific contribution to dental in helping dentists not only get into private practice successfully but outpace the competition."

-Alex Nudel, Founder, Revenuewell

"Just as there are specialists in dental care, there are people that specialize in helping dentists start up and build their practices. Building a trusted team of people that understand your specific goals and needs, and leveraging their expertise will give you the resources needed to achieve your goals. I have seen the professional guidance that Fortune Management provides to help doctors avoid pitfalls that cost time, money, and headaches and will maximize potential for success!"

-Andrew Kaltenbach, Regional Sales Manager, A-dec Inc.

"Starting a new business is hard. Starting a dental office from scratch is harder. As a dentist, I quickly realized that everyone wanted a piece of the pie. And I yearned for a trusted advisor. Someone who had experience, was practice savvy, and who was unabashedly my advocate. I found that and more with Jonathan

and Fortune Management. Their attention to detail, their persistence and perseverance during the toughest stretches of the game, and the relationship they built which allowed us to celebrate our successes together have left me a fan for life. They are my magic wand and I am so so happy I have them in my corner."

-Dr. Amisha Singh, Smile Always Dental

"Through the help of Fortune Management, I was able to find an opportunity that was meant for me. Jonathan always took time to address my concerns, sort available options, and eased my stress while still working multiple jobs! He is easy to talk to and his diversified background will be an asset to anyone he helps. I am sincerely grateful to have had someone looking out in my best interest during the entire process. Thank you Jonathan and Fortune for the continual support."

-Dr. Darcy Kasner, Artisan Dentistry

"One thing most associates are feared of is opening a startup. In fact I was a lot nervous too. With your help throughout the process, today my practice is up and running full-time smoothly for almost 4 months. Now I realize how one bad decision in the process could have impacted my startup badly. I have been recommending you to all my friends who are in process of making those decisions. Your help during every step, be it planning, construction, equipment bidding, hiring and most importantly marketing helped me open office on time by staying within my planned budget. It was a long process and whenever I was stressed, calling you and talking to you made me feel much better. You always boosted good confidence in me. You were my 911 throughout the process.

Now that my office project is over for you, I truly hope that I have a privilege to call you my friend."

-Dr. Pritpal Gill, Oak Dentistry

FORTUNE MANAGEMENT

Fortune Management is an organization committed to helping doctors and their teams turn their dreams into realities. We believe in the best balance of practice management and personal development, to create not only the structure but, more important, the culture to create an extraordinary practice and an extraordinary life for the people who work within the profession and for the patients they serve.

Fortune Management is made up of over 100 Executive Coaches across the nation to provide a first class experience to the clients we serve. Our coaches represent three distinct roles for clients in our network; An Executive Coach, a Practice Management Specialist, and a Key Business Strategist.

The Role of an Executive Coach:

Fortune Management is very adamant that our core difference is being a coach to our clients, not a consultant. We find out what the doctor or owner wants and help them achieve it. We firmly believe it is not our job to put our expectations on our clients. We hold our clients accountable for what they want and their actions and decisions that bring them closer to their ultimate vision.

The Role of a Practice Management Specialist:

This means implementing key practice management systems that address the five engines of the business or practice; sales/marketing, technology, clinical, organization, and financial, all focused around the practice's vision. We make sure that the practice runs as an efficient, profitable business with or without the owner.

The Role of a Key Business Strategist:

This means working on fulfilling the doctor's vision for his business to achieve his vision for life. We help our clients act like a CEO and make educated, sophisticated business decisions that will advance them in their career. This could involve mergers and acquisitions, bringing on associates that are future business partners, adding multiple locations, real estate purchases, bringing in specialists to create a multi-specialty practice, remodeling their current facility to create their dream practice and so much more.